FAMILY BASED TREATMENT IN COMMUNICATIVE DISORDERS

A SYSTEMIC APPROACH

JAMES R. ANDREWS, Ph.D.
Professor
Department of Communicative Disorders
Northern Illinois University
DeKalb, Illinois

MARY A. ANDREWS, M.S.
Instructor
Department of Communicative Disorders
Northern Illinois University
DeKalb, Illinois
&
Couple and Family Therapist
Kairos Family Center
Elgin, Illinois

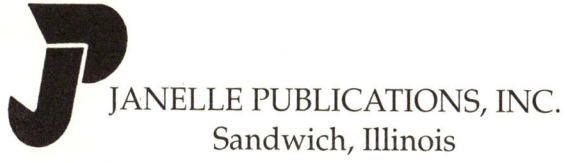

JANELLE PUBLICATIONS, INC.
Sandwich, Illinois

Copyright © 1990, Janelle Publications, Inc.,
625 West Church Street, Sandwich, Illinois 60548

All rights reserved. No part of this book may be reproduced in any form or by any means, including photocopying, recording, or used by any information storage and retrieval system, without permission in writing from the Publisher.

Printed in the United States of America.
ISBN 0-9626939-0-1

CONTENTS

Prologue v

Acknowledgements vii

Introduction 1

Chapter 1 5
The Systemic Perspective

Chapter 2 23
Eliciting and Maintaining Cooperation

Chapter 3 29
Convening the Family

Chapter 4 37
Sharing an Understanding of the Problem

Chapter 5 49
Agreeing on Changes and Setting Goals

Chapter 6 61
Assignments

Chapter 7 71
Assessing Treatment Effectiveness

Chapter 8 84
Termination and Linkage

Chapter 9 89
Counseling Techniques

Chapter 10 117
Application to Early Childhood
Speech, Language and Hearing Problems

Chapter 11 155
Application to Families with Middle Childhood
and Adolescent Children

Chapter 12 175
Application to Adults and Their Families

Bibliography 193

Index 201

PROLOGUE

The Andrews must be congratulated for the first organized approach to utilization of families in the speech-language therapeutic process. As healthcare costs and educational costs soar, our profession like many others, is being encouraged to develop and adopt more efficient and cost effective methods of treatment. In the public schools, collaborative teaching methods are being adopted on experimental bases in many districts. In the private sector, speech-language pathologists, occupational therapists, and physical therapists are finding rehabilitation resources more and more limited. The latter has resulted in patients being discharged to homes or extended care facilities much sooner than in the past, thus placing new demands and treatment responsibility on families and nursing staff.

There is great pressure on all of the "one-on-one" clinical practitioners to find less costly avenues for maximizing change in our clients. What could facilitate the therapeutic process more efficiently than utilizing resources of family, friends, or institutional staff? These persons are frequently very eager to help. But, as important, they provide the possibility of hours of "realistic" interactions with the client for each single visit by a professional. If I were asked to pay for any clinical services for my child, husband, or parent, I would opt for Family Based Treatment.

Just reading the Andrews' book has made me feel empowered as a partner in many aspects of problem solving within my own family. How exciting it must be for their clients to feel this same confidence in working to change the speech or language deficits of a loved one. And how rewarding it must be for the families to share in the success.

The Andrews' Family Based Treatment suddenly seems long overdue. I suspect it will lead the way in developing more pragmatic and efficient avenues for speech and language habilitation that utilize family, friends, and allied health professionals.

Martha S. Burns, Ph.D.
April, 1990

ACKNOWLEDGEMENTS

We could not have had better teachers than the families with whom we have worked. We gratefully acknowledge their contribution to the development of a model in which they are an integral part. They showed us how to include them as full participants in treatment as we joined together in search of change.

The support and encouragement of the faculty and staff of the Department of Communicative Disorders, Northern Illinois University, is also very much appreciated. They actively supported us even when we commandeered the best and largest room (the Bruce Irvin Suite) in the Speech and Hearing Clinic (families don't fit into the small treatment rooms characteristic of university clinics)! Their honest and legitimate questioning, as well as that of our students, helps us continue to refine the model.

Finally, since this book is about families, we must say a word about our own. Our children Dave, Tim, and Mark have taught us about families in a remarkably creative manner. They understand that parents as well as children participate in a developmental journey and continue to show us, in many fascinating ways, the power of the family.

INTRODUCTION

This book is written for speech-language pathologists and audiologists who want to include family members in treatment. Many human service professionals have an instinctive sense that families offer rich resources and that it is impractical to provide services without family participation. If this is your orientation, we offer this book for your evaluation and enjoyment. If you have not yet reached the conclusion that families add the missing element, we offer this book for your consideration and contemplation. If you find new ideas thought-provoking, challenging, and stimulating, we offer this book for your critical deliberation and pleasure.

The clinical approach to be described is based on a systemic rather than a linear paradigm. Professionals who use a systemic model attend to the continually evolving transactions that occur between people. Individual change is facilitated by change in the system. Those who use a linear model, on the other hand, focus on cause-effect relationships and change is expected and assessed only within the individual. The assumptions of the linear (individual) model are so pervasive in speech-language pathology and audiology and taken so much for granted by all of us that it is likely to take time and practice to make the shift to a systemic way of thinking. Essentially every book, every clinical procedure, every assessment tool, and every physical setting in which we practice assumes that the clinician offers services that are based on a linear model. In this respect, this book is "news of a difference" (Bateson, 1979), to use a phrase familiar to family therapists. It "announces" that there is another way of thinking about what we do. We are still in the process of shifting to a systemic paradigm, and it is likely that most people who read this book will find that that shift takes time and intentionality. For many, the effort will not only be exciting, but rewarding in that an expanse of new clinical options becomes available and opportunities for change outside the parameters of the traditional individual model will be discovered.

The book is also different from many books in the field because it it is written out of our clinical experience. Families have taught us how to connect theory with practice and we attempt to pass this information on to the reader through descriptions and examples. Several innovative family therapists have influenced our work and the contribution of their thinking and practice to the development of the Family Based Treatment model is acknowledged. deShazer (1985), Fisch, Weakland, and Segal (1982), Keeney (1983), Minuchin (1974), O'Hanlon and Weiner-Davis (1989), and Tomm (1984, 1988) have been significant influences. The influence of Haley (1987) will be particularly evident to the reader who is familiar with his problem solving model.

The approach described in this book is offered as a supplement or alternative to the traditional individual model of speech-language-hearing treatment services. Not everyone who wants to work with families practices in a setting which permits this to the extent that we describe it. Few, if any, will do it exactly in the manner that we do. It is expected that the approach will be adapted to the reader's clinical situation and that selected parts of the process and some of the techniques will be used as the reader relates to families in the manner most appropriate and feasible. In some settings, perhaps it will be possible to select one family and involve the members more completely in treatment. In others, some of the principles and techniques may be used in parent conferences. In yet others, family members who previously sat in the waiting room may be invited into the treatment room with the clinician. Frankly, we do not believe that anyone who has a desire to work with families could read this book and not do something different in the way he/she practices the profession.

The style of this book is personal and to some extent isomorphic to the way we work with families. In that vein, a brief description of how we started inviting family participation might be useful. We began working with families in a university speech and hearing clinic eight years ago. Mary had, and still has, a private practice as a family therapist. In that practice she received more than the expected number of referrals of families who were dealing with family problems

Introduction

exacerbated by disability. When these families were referred for family therapy, their children were often adolescents. Typical problems included disempowered parents, dysfunctional family communication, socially unacceptable adolescent behavior, and difficulty launching the young adult. Problems that might have been effectively confronted when the child was young had developed into emotionally laden challenges that left parents feeling impotent and discouraged. Interactions between families and professionals, in most cases, were no more satisfying than interactions among family members. Parents showed alienation from the social service system and most professionals labeled the families as uncooperative. Mary hypothesized that many of these problems could have been prevented had families been members of the habilitative team from the outset. At the same time, Jim was teaching classes, supervising clinical services, and becoming increasingly involved in parenting three young children. Parenting his own children gave Jim a new appreciation for family interaction which influenced the way he taught and supervised. Rather, for example, than have parents sit in the waiting room of the clinic, he asked them to come into the observation or treatment room with him. He suggested to students that during assessments family members remain in the room and participate at some level. Interviews of parents took on a new look as information they offered became more highly valued than in the past.

    It was from this perspective that we decided to combine our expertise and interests and to work together. We have worked with families of all ages and with many types of communicative disorders. This work has been supported by our colleagues and students at Northern Illinois University and the result is a new and different approach to the treatment of communicative disorders. We call this new approach Family Based Treatment.

CHAPTER 1

THE SYSTEMIC PERSPECTIVE

Family members can be a significant resource for change. Speech-language pathologists and audiologists, knowing this, have made various attempts over the years to include parents in treatment. These efforts, however, have nearly always been based on the assumptions and framework of the linear (individual) treatment model. Mothers, for example, have been enlisted to carry out structured therapy plans, in effect, assuming the role of an aide working under strict supervision of the speech-language pathologist. The individual continues to be the unit of treatment in this case, but the treatment plan is implemented by someone other than the clinician. More routinely, speech-language pathologists attempt to extend their influence by asking family members to practice words, sentences, etc. with clients much in the same way that physicians give prescriptions to patients. Compliance with the speech-language pathologist's assignments becomes an issue in some cases and families may be cast in the role of being "uncooperative." Other attempts to involve families are educational in nature. Family members are told about speech-language and hearing problems to inform them about the nature of these disorders. Brochures are available to describe aphasia, cleft palate, language delay, stuttering, and other communicative disorders. All of these efforts are logical and useful extensions of services offered within a linear model. Within that approach, the most significant changes in communicative behavior occur during sessions with the speech-language pathologist. These changes may be enhanced by family cooperation and understanding but participation of families is secondary to the role of the professional.

While the traditional model continues to be satisfactory in some clinical situations, a desire to enlarge the focus of treatment beyond the direct efforts of speech-language pathologists is emerging. Frassinelli, et al. (1983), Garbee (1982), Manolson (1985), Neidecker (1987), Superior & Lelchook (1986), and Williams (1986), for example, have suggested that the responsibility for changing communicative behavior may be shared with other significant people in clients' lives and that change might occur more rapidly and efficiently if this were done. Further, the importance of family participation is magnified when we think of offering services to infants and toddlers for whom the traditional individual model seems particularly inappropriate. Federal law (P.L. 99-457) even assures that families will participate in services offered to this population.

Changes in treatment approaches which go beyond variations of the individual model have been slow to occur on a widespread basis. This, we believe, is in large part due to the fact that the assumptions underlying the individual direct services model of treatment are incompatible with services that are collaborative in nature. We believe that effective use of the resources of families (or of other professional persons) requires a systemic rather than an individual perspective. The individual model, however, is so firmly in place that it has continued to be the perspective from which involvement of families and others is understood by most clinicians. A shift to a systemic understanding of treatment may be a prerequisite to involving families and/or other professionals successfully in the habilitation/rehabilitation process.

A PARADIGM SHIFT

In order to successfully involve families in the therapy process it is necessary for the clinician to change from a

The Systemic Perspective

linear to a systemic way of *thinking* about treatment. This change in thinking may be referred to as a paradigm shift. As the clinician's view is altered in the direction of systemic thinking, a changed perception affects the manner in which his/her professional expertise is used. For example, as the clinician begins to view the interactions between a client and one or more of the client's family members as critical to the assessment and treatment of speech-language-hearing disorders, the clinician will then want to invite those family members to participate in the assessment and treatment process in an active manner.

The changes in thinking that impact the way the clinician conducts therapy are a shift from one "truth" to "many truths," from an either/or orientation to a both/and orientation, from labeling behaviors to identifying interactive patterns, from a problem-focus to a solution-focus, and from linear cause-effect change to systems transformation.

From One Truth to Many Truths

The phrase "polyocular view" has been used by deShazer (1985) to describe a situation in which many different interpretations of the same phenomenon are received and accepted as true. The combined resources of many eyes (polyocular) generate a view that offers more options for change than that of the one-eyed perspective. Similarly, sound (music in particular) takes on a new dimension as several tracks are superimposed to create a relational whole that is different from the sound generated by one track alone. The sound tracks may be complimentary or dissonant when combined but each by itself is an accurate representation of its own tune.

Each of the people who interact with the individual having a speech-language disorder has a view of the problem that is influenced by the particular perspective of that person as well as by the way in which his/her observations/interactions affect the phenomenon under consideration. One of the language delayed children that we treated was seen as stubborn by his mother, mechanically gifted by his father, cute by his grandfather, autistic by a school psychologist, retarded by his teacher, and language impaired by a speech-language pathologist. Each of these views, though different, was correct from the perspective of the person expressing a "truth." Many factors, of course, influenced each view including the professional, personal, and family relationship of each person to the child. The clinician must honestly view all these perspectives as accurate *when considered from the point of view of the person expressing the opinion*. This understanding will assist the clinician in developing a systemic assessment of the problem to be treated.

From Either/Or to Both/And

The polyocular view naturally requires that the clinician adopt a both/and orientation. This is the idea that two or more beliefs, assessments, or observations, though different can be correct. For example, if in a family the mother is very structured, organized and concrete in her view of child rearing and requires orderly behavior from her children while father is playful, relaxed, and spontaneous with few structured expectations, the children are doubly fortunate because two very useful styles are being modeled and encouraged. This both/and view of two different parenting styles releases resources that will enhance the children's development. If, however, an either/or orientation is adopted by the parents (and children) they are likely to challenge one another about the correctness of each perspective. This challenge will result in a conflict that is likely to banish one of the parenting "truths" to a covert position in the family's relational style. This either/or conflict diminishes the range of options that are available to those fortunate families that adopt a both/and perspective.

When the clinician adopts a polyocular view, which includes a both/and orientation, he/she realizes that the professional perspective regarding treatment is as correct as each family member's view of the problem. An important variable must be added, however. In a family, parents need to accept responsibility for organizing differences so that family life is enhanced. The parents may need to choose situations that are more appropriate for orderly control than for spontaneous play and teach these differences to their children. Or, one parent may need to approach the other in order to discuss these differences and reach concensus about how to manage them. The possibilities are numerous and the both/and view requires friendly cooperation in order to facilitate optimum use of different yet valid opinions. In like manner, the professional must accept responsibility for organizing the variety of views expressed so that the treatment climate is enhanced. This is usually done through friendly discussion of the differences expressed and by deciding which viewpoints can be most effectively accessed for change to occur.

From Labeling Behaviors to Identifying Interactive Patterns

The clinician, when meeting a client and his/her family members for the first time, usually wants to make a diagnosis so that treatment goals can be established. Generally, the speech-language behavior is described in behavioral terms and a label is given to the problem. Sometimes this diagnosis is easily determined as in most cases of adult stuttering. At other times, the diagnosis is more elusive, particularly when the clinician is confronted with language delay, apraxic-like articulation errors, or mixed functional-organic communicative disorders.

When the diagnosis is clear and is agreed upon by everyone present, the systemic clinician begins immediately to explore the interactive patterns in which the speech-language difficulty is embedded. When the diagnosis is elusive, or several different diagnoses are offered, it is wise for the clinician to abandon his/her efforts to find a "label" and, instead, begin to explore interactive patterns in order to gather more data about the problem. Ultimately, as the clinician conducts this exploration the need for a label diminishes in importance. When a diagnosis must be put on paper because this is required of the clinician, he/she realizes that the label is often a metaphor for the problem which may in fact have no useful name.

Consider a family that includes a fifteen year old daughter. On a particular day in January this girl's behavior is labeled by mother as "grouchy" and by grandma as "sullen." Her boyfriend says she's "upset" and her girlfriend worries that she's "depressed." Each of these labels is interesting and is viewed as true by the person expressing concern, but is of limited usefulness in exploring possible solutions to the discomfort shown by the teenager. If a friend of mother asks questions such as, "How does daughter show you her 'grouchiness'?"; "What do you do in response?"; "Who else seems to notice that daughter is upset?"; and "How does this person respond?" the mother and friend begin to uncover events which place the "grouchiness" in an interactive context. This interactive understanding of "grouchy behavior" will lead to possibilities for change more efficiently than will the acceptance of the label, "grouchy."

Similarly, when the clinician adopts a systemic perspective, he/she shifts the focus from a primary concern for finding a label to an exploration of the interactive nature of the problem. Questions such as, "How does Timmy let you know what he wants?"; "How do you respond when this happens?"; "Who else seems to be concerned?"; "How does that person respond?"; and "What's happening during the times when Timmy communicates best?" open the discussion to interactive exploration. The clinician, client, and family members may then begin to discover new possibilities for change. (A detailed description of the use of questions in exploring interactive patterns is found in Chapter 9.)

From a Problem Focus to a Solution Focus

When the clinician, client, and family explore the

interactive events that surround a communicative disorder, the focus of treatment moves in the direction of solutions. Sometimes new solutions are created. Often, solutions are already a part of the client's and family's behavioral repertoire and simply need to be unearthed and actuated by the clinician.

In one of the author's family therapy practice, for example, a family was very concerned because their fourteen year old son was "lazy." Exploration of the problem revealed that this "laziness" was shown most clearly during times the son was supposed to be doing homework. Further exploration revealed that there were many times when the son did not show "laziness" but showed behaviors that his parents labeled "responsible" and "energetic." These behaviors were associated with his basketball playing, snacking, and guitar playing. Since it was determined that the boy was not a "lazy boy," but one who needed to learn to show his responsible and energetic behavior in another area of his life, the focus of the family shifted toward helping him apply these skills to homework completion. When the family shifted their view to a solution focus, this freed the boy to recognize and use his abilities differently.

Similarly, as the clinician shifts his/her focus toward uncovering and creating solutions, the clinician and the family are likely to find unexpected resources that can be used to treat the speech-language-hearing problem. While exploring the interaction surrounding language delayed behavior for example, the parents and clinician may discover that there are times when the child does use words. At these times the parents may notice that they are speaking calmly and slowly to one another, that they are relaxed, and that they are less likely to ask the child questions or ask the child to name things. These behaviors may be partial solutions to changing the environmental context of the low verbal child. When focused on solutions, the systemic clinician creates a climate that facilitates change in clients with communicative disorders.

The boy who is seen as "responsible" instead of "lazy" is more likely to do his homework. The parents who are seen as "sensitive" and "creative" are more likely to be successful in helping their family member who is communicatively disordered than those who are viewed as "uncaring" and "inept." When the clinician adopts a solution focus, greater use can be made of the positive resources available within the family system (O'Hanlon & Weiner-Davis, (1989).

From Cause-Effect Change to System Transformation

Most clinicians think of change in a cause-effect way. For example, the clinician first identifies a problem such as: "articulation of speech was limited to bilabial, tongue tip-alveolar, and glottal sounds. The latter place of articulation was overused with glottal stops being substituted for many voiceless consonants" (Andrews & Andrews, 1986a, p. 410). With this assessment in mind, goals are set and treatment proceeds. Usually there seems to be a direct cause-effect relationship between changes in the client's speech and the clinician's implementation of specific treatment strategies. However, many clients report other unexpected changes that seem to be related to the speech-language change, but cannot be linked to the treatment process in a linear cause-effect way. Changes such as "he's talking more," "he's more demanding," and "he stands up for himself" are typical of those reported by clients and/or their family members but are not specifically related to treatment efforts to "eliminate the use of glottal stops being substituted for many voiceless consonants." The clinician, client, and family sense, however, that these behavioral changes are associated with the speech-language treatment process. These changes may be said to result from a "system transformation" (Tomm, 1984).

When working with families, the clinician will experience both system transformations and cause-effect changes. As the speech-language-hearing difficulty is assessed and as the family is respectfully included in that process, the family is likely to transform itself in ways that cannot always be predicted by the clinician. Often these changes are unexpected and are directly related to speech-language improvement.

As we worked with T. (age 4), his mother, father, and three siblings, we and the family decided together to use the family's resources to help T. become more intelligible (Andrews & Andrews, 1986a). After fourteen sessions over a nine month period, T.'s intelligibility had improved nearly 100% and our services were terminated. During that process, the family had transformed itself in many surprising ways. Formerly, they had been labeled by the professional community as "uncooperative" because they were failing to keep appointments and not following through with treatment recommendations. Near the end of Family Based Treatment, T.'s kindergarten teacher reported that he looked different, was more kempt, and that his mother had become interested in his work and was eager to cooperate with classroom goals. His formerly unintelligible speech was reported to be completely intelligible in every context. This was confirmed by his second grade teacher, two years later, when she expressed surprise when informed that T. had once had a speech problem. Other changes occurred which likely continue to reverberate in the family system in unexpected and surprising ways.

None of these changes could be linked in a linear fashion to a specific cause. Even the speech-language change could not be specifically linked to our work with the family nor could the change be specifically linked to the competent, involved mother, or the quiet, controlled father, or the teasing brothers, or the nurturing sister. The family had transformed itself in a way that was coherent with their idiosyncratic style (Dell, 1982) and these changes had impacted many areas of T.'s life.

It would have been very difficult to study the 28 sets of interactions occurring amongst the eight people involved in treatment. Even if this were possible, the reductionist view of "what happened" could not fully reveal the systemic transformations that occurred in a co-evolutionary manner over time. Rather, the family system was accessed in a way that freed its members to take charge of change in their own idiosyncratic way. This included their desire to use the expertise of the clinicians who worked with them.

FAMILY BASED TREATMENT

Family Based Treatment involves the entire family in all aspects of assessment and treatment. The family, rather than the individual, is viewed as the unit of treatment. Family interactive patterns that facilitate change are discussed, rewarded, and amplified; family members become equal partners with the professional as members of the rehabilitation team; and counseling is an integral part of the assessment and treatment process.

Unit of Treatment

When the individual is the unit of treatment, the context for assessment and rehabilitative services is the client-clinician dyad. The communicative disorder is understood and treated as it occurs in that setting. As such, the speech-language problem is viewed as a static condition of the individual even though the client may experience variations in different situations and the clinician understands that these may occur. The problem, however, is seldom actually seen by the clinician in other contexts for purposes of additional evaluation and treatment. Treatment is limited to time spent with the speech-language pathologist and carryover of new behaviors into other situations is accepted as a potential problem.

When the family is the unit of treatment, the context for assessment, treatment services, and change is the family-clinician system. Communication is evaluated and understood as it is manifested, shaped, and reacted to in the interactions of the family. Treatment occurs in the natural, functional environment of the family and carryover is not an issue since the clinician assists the family to effect change within real-life interactive situations. Family interactive patterns in which the communicative disorder is embedded may also be observed. This gives the clinician a greater depth of understanding of the problem and increases options for change.

Role of the Professional

In the individual model, treatment decisions are made by the professional and the client; family members are expected to comply with the habilitative plan. Consequently, when outside assignments are not completed, when the client arrives late for sessions, or the client appears disinterested, the client and/or family are said to be uncooperative.

In a Family Based Treatment model the family becomes part of the solution and a member of the habilitative team. Family members participate in the assessment; have input as to the goals of treatment; and, with the help of the speech-language pathologist, utilize their resources to change the communicative behavior of their own family member. Compliance is not an issue when families participate at this level because each family's style of cooperating is accessed and reinforced by the clinician.

Use of Counseling

Traditionally, information supplements the treatment process and counseling is of an informative nature. The clinician attempts to help the client and/or family members understand what he/she is doing in treatment sessions and why this is important. The clinician typically uses professional language and attempts to teach the family to understand the problem in the same manner as it is understood by the clinician.

In a Family Based Treatment model, counseling is integrated with assessment and treatment. Counseling techniques are used by the clinician to promote family participation, to respond to attitudes and feelings that accompany disability, and to accomplish the tasks associated with each step of the Family Based Treatment process. Counseling skills are integrated into the entire rehabilitative process. The clinician builds upon the family's perspective of the problem to lead the family to a greater understanding of the communicative disorder and how it may be changed. Intentionally adding to the family's understanding, rather than ignoring it, is a necessary step for full family participation.

FOUR SYSTEMIC PRINCIPLES

Four systemic principles provide a rationale for the Family Based Treatment model. First, *one part of the family cannot be understood in isolation from the rest of the system* (Epstein & Bishop, 1981). The behavior of each family member may be understood more completely when it is interpreted relative to the patterns, beliefs, and customs of the family as a whole than when it is analyzed in isolation. Most everyone has had the experience of gaining insights into the behavior of a friend upon being introduced to that person's family of origin. Behaviors of the individual are understood differently in that context. It is traditional in our society for young couples anticipating a serious relationship to meet one another's families. We can assume that many insights have been gleaned through such meetings. While the ostensible purpose may be for the family to meet and evaluate the offspring's friend, the larger amount of information and perhaps the greater evaluation may fall to the "intended" upon seeing the potential mate in the interactive environment of his/her family of origin.

Similarly, the details of a communicative disorder may be comprehended in a different way when the clinician views the client in the environment of his/her family than when evaluating and treating the individual alone. In the family context the communicative behavior of the client may be observed relative to the interactions of the entire system. Some families with whom we have worked have had one or two members who were very articulate and verbal and the child with a language delay had few opportunities to talk. In other cases, family members were so quiet and independent that the child with a language delay, like the rest of the family, rarely sought or received interactive attention. We are not suggesting that there is anything "wrong" with these or other interactive behaviors we have observed in families, nor do we discuss what we observe with families in other than a neutral and accepting manner. Given a communicative disorder, however, those interactive patterns that appear to be facilitative of change may be reinforced and expanded and those that seem to be perpetuating the problem may be discussed and altered. The information that contextual observation yields is rich not only for describing the problem but for developing interventions for change.

Second, *the parts of a family are interrelated; change in one part influences change in other parts of the system* (Epstein & Bishop, 1981). Most everyone who is part of a family has experienced the results of one person being sick with the flu and incapacitated for a day or two. The effects of even a temporary illness such as this are not limited to the person who is ill; everyone in the family is affected. The specific manner in which the lives of the different family members are touched varies with idiosyncratic family patterns, the roles of family members, and the developmental stage of the family. It is not difficult to imagine the varying effects of illness to a father, mother, or young child in a family with preschool and school-age children. While the specifics are different, it is no less a matter of reacting when one member of a senior citizen couple is ill. When one member of a family is out of town, in trouble, happy, depressed, angry, etc. the behavior of everyone else in the family is influenced and everyone reacts in some way. One needs only to consider different situations in his/her own family to appreciate the complex nature of overt and covert reactions and interactions that might accompany a change in one individual.

Similarly, when one member of a family has a communicative disorder, the behavior of all other family members is affected and all members react. Some typical reactions we have observed include asking the adult with aphasia many questions; asking a child to name pictures and objects; showing anger and embarrassment over a family member's speech disorder; rewarding the verbalizations of a child with delayed language; helping the person with a head injury by saying the words he appeared to be wanting to say; and exaggerating the consonants for the young child with a repaired cleft palate. Obviously, some family reactions facilitate desirable change more than others. When family members of a young child who stuttered modified their behavior to ask fewer questions and reduce the amount of educational instruction they were providing, the child's ability to control his fluency increased. In another family, inattentiveness combined with very limited communicative attempts by the child were part of a family interactive system in which mom and nine year old daughter both talked a lot while dad was extremely quiet. When the verbal output of the two more talkative family members was reduced, both the child and his father began to speak more. When family members are an integral part of assessment and treatment and have techniques for reinforcing appropriate communicative behavior, services are not limited to time spent with the clinician and carryover is enhanced from the outset (Andrews & Andrews, 1986b).

    Family members also react to speech-language improvement of their members. The brothers and sisters of a child with unintelligible speech described him as "meaner" and "bossy" after his intelligibility improved and he spoke more. His parents interpreted this behavior as "standing up for himself" and as showing assertiveness verbally rather than physically (Andrews & Andrews, 1986a). The parents of this same child were reported by other social service professionals to be more cooperative. The teacher indicated that the child was dressed better at school and had more friends, and his parents reported that his grades improved. Many changes accompanied an improvement in this child's speech intelligibility.

    When a communicative disorder is associated with permanent disability, the effects of that disability extend beyond the daily activities of the immediate family members. Grandparents, great-grandparents, and all extended family members are affected by the disability in ways that permeate their lives throughout the life span. The disability may be known at birth, may become known as the child matures, or may occur later in the life of the individual. Each family member and professional working with the client is profoundly affected by this unexpected event or change.

Third, *transactional patterns of the family shape the behavior of family members* (Epstein & Bishop, 1981). Every individual is affected by the immediate and long ranging family events that shape and form the life experience. The pull of the family system is felt by clinicians and clients alike as they work for speech-language improvement. The speech-language pathologist's awareness of some of these influences may be used to help families promote change in their member who is communicatively disordered. Some of these transactional patterns can be observed by attending to interactions during family sessions; others can be accessed through careful questioning and tracking of behavioral sequences. Some are revealed over time as family members and the clinician become better acquainted; others will remain unknown both to the family and to the clinician.

Complex interactions related to a speech-language problem are likely to include both verbal and non-verbal repetitive patterns among family members. For example, the noisy messy eating of a dysarthric teenager evoked admonitions and advice from his mother. Younger brother reacted to the conversation by becoming silent and dad responded to all of this with anger at both his wife and the teenager. The teenager in turn ate faster and, therefore, messier and noisier. This pattern, according to the family, repeated itself nearly everyday at dinnertime. The pattern was changed by a combination of experimentation with different eating techniques and the use of counseling techniques which helped the family view the problem in a different way. It is not uncommon for speech-language-hearing problems to be embedded in family interactive patterns. In another case, a child with a language delay phonated; mom imitated the vocalization;

the child repeated the utterance; and both mom and dad cheered, smiled, patted the child, and showed pleasure in general. This was a pattern which we rewarded and, with the help of the parents, amplified. In a different family, a typical pattern was for mom to say a word and then ask the child to say it. The child ignored mom's repeated urgings, dad showed annoyance with the child, mom tried harder to encourage the child to say the word to no avail, and the child walked away. Mom then defended the child to dad by saying something positive about him and dad responded with a look of disgust or displeasure. With both parent's help, this pattern was changed by finding a more effective way for mom to encourage the child to speak. When the child responded appropriately this successful interaction was discussed with dad.

Fourth, *a family's structure, organization, and developmental stage are important factors in determining the behavior of family members* (Epstein & Bishop, 1981). Every family undergoes developmental changes over time, has a hierarchical structure, and adopts certain roles that are fulfilled by individual family members. Rules about the family's organization of these roles are often covert but are usually accepted and understood by each family member. For example, in a two parent family with two young children and a grandmother living with the family (structure), the roles may be traditional in that father is the primary breadwinner, mother the primary caregiver, and the grandmother a respected but peripheral family member (roles). This family will organize itself around these roles with the parents assuming responsibility for managing the lives of the children (hierarchy). While the clinician may believe that the father should be more involved than he is, the right of the family to organize itself must be respected. It would be inappropriate, for example, to assign the uninvolved father to read stories to the communicatively disordered child. It would, however, be appropriate to honestly determine who usually would do such an activity and the circumstances under which it could be done and to enlist father's support as mother or grandmother carried out the task. As a family evolves over time, changes in society, family structure, and capabilities of the children will result in developmental changes necessitating different types of assignments. Learning about how families organize themselves can be beneficial to the clinician who wishes to capitalize on this information in order to give meaningful assignments to family members. When a child is not talking, for example, the parents usually are aware of those techniques that are and are not successful in eliciting language. They know the child's reactions to different situations, when the time is appropriate to use an intervention, and when it is not. They also know the particular types of interactions with which each family member will be most successful. Further, while some families like to look at books, others like to play on the floor, or mother likes to look at books with the children, but father prefers active play. In some families father's role is to be supportive of mother rather than to actually intervene in any active way. In other families, grandmother may play an important role in child care, or stepparents may be actively involved with the child who has a communicative disorder.

As the clinician shows an understanding of the different family developmental stages, a respect for the family's structure, and an interest in the way the family assigns and organizes roles, he/she will be able to give assignments to family members that fit their individual strengths and styles.

SUMMARY

Speech-language pathology services are steeped in the tradition of the individual medical model of service delivery. Efforts to include families and other professionals in clinical services have arisen out of assumptions associated with the traditional individual model. A systemic rather than a linear paradigm seems necessary in order to effectively expand the influence of speech-language services through including families and others in treatment. The systemic model requires a shift in thinking about human behavior and an understanding of systems principles.

Family Based treatment is a systemic approach to clinical services in which families are involved in all aspects of assessment and treatment. The model offers both a theoretical framework and a process for providing services in the family context. Some general principles of cooperation, also necessary for successful family participation in treatment, will be discussed in Chapter 2.

CHAPTER 2

ELICITING AND MAINTAINING COOPERATION

The attitude of the professional toward the family is critical for eliciting family cooperation and participation. The speech-language pathologist or audiologist who genuinely believes that families have valuable resources for creating change and who encourages families to use these resources is likely to be successful in gaining the cooperation of family members as full participants in treatment. In Family Based Treatment the clinician seeks as many ways as possible to access the resources of the family as well as those of the member with the handicap.

When the individual is the unit of treatment it is customary to seek a level of rapport with the client. Probably everyone involved with students has seen lesson plans where the only goal was "to gain rapport" or its corollary, "to get to know the client." Most of us neither spend an hour on this goal alone nor assume that it can be completely accomplished in one session. We do, however, have a sense that it is important for clients to have a positive regard for us, and us for them, in order to gain their cooperation and thereby elicit change. It is no less important to seek a level of rapport with families when they are the unit of treatment. No one would show disrespect for a client or give the impression that he/she is not good enough to change, yet, inadvertently, this is the signal that families sometimes receive from members of helping professions. Under these circumstances, families may devalue their resources and lose confidence in their ability to participate effectively in services.

The following guidelines serve as reminders for us as much as for the reader. They were developed out of our experience in working with families and teaching the Family Based Treatment model in classes and workshops.

Respond to Family Members' Expertise

Families cooperate most when they are acknowledged as experts about their own members and when their viewpoints are sought and appreciated. A family knows more about its member with a disability than anyone else. Combining the expertise of a family with that of the clinician can result in a powerful force for change. Families *assume* the expertise of the speech-language pathologist; that aspect of the relationship is a given. The speech-language pathologist, however, must overtly acknowledge the expertise of families and assure them that the information they offer is valuable. Since this acknowledgement is not necessarily part of the typical family-professional relationship, family members may need to be convinced that their expertise is desired.

Acknowledge Family Members' Emotions

Families cooperate most when they are allowed to express emotions and feelings about their family members in an empathic atmosphere. Not all professionals are comfortable in the presence of a client or family member who is discouraged, crying, or angry. It is not difficult to show in many nonverbal ways as well as through verbal responses that emotions of distress are not welcome. This may even be the most efficient way to conduct individual treatment sessions. When family members are involved, however, strong emotions are likely to be expressed from time to time. It is normal for family members to react to disability. Responses from the clinician that are most helpful are those that restate or reflect the feelings being expressed. These skills are discussed in Chapter 9. Responses that are least helpful are those that give advice, attempt to encourage the person or to cheer him/her up, minimize the problem, change the subject, or seek more facts. It is natural for families to reveal feelings when they participate in the treatment process. In many cases, after expressing emotions in an atmosphere of acceptance and understanding, the family shows renewed energy and an increased appreciation for the family-clinician relationship.

Respect Family Members' Concerns

Families cooperate most when their very strong concerns about their member who is disabled are viewed objectively and empathically. Many of the families with whom we work have sought services which seemed unnecessary or even useless to us. Angela, a three year old with mental retardation, was treated by a chiropractor in hopes that spinal adjustments would help her. Gina, age six with autistic-like behavior, began a program of patterned limb motion and eye exercises because her parents thought it might improve her behavior. Tom, fifteen years old and cerebral palsied, had his tongue clipped and underwent massive orthodontia in hopes that his tongue would move better if it had more room. These are just a few examples of the efforts of families to help their children. In no case was our opinion sought. These families wanted to help their children, not discuss rationales or hear professional disagreements. If our opinion had been asked we would have given it. Since it was not, we attempted to join the families in their concern for the family member and desire to do everything possible. Responding to the emotions that led to their decision, joining them in their desire for change, using neutral questions (see Chapter 9) to learn more about the supplementary services, and using the services in a positive way all seemed more likely to be effective than showing skepticism or questioning the family's judgment.

Allow Family Imperfection

Families cooperate most when the clinician recognizes and encourages their ability to change and accepts that families will not do everything perfectly. Most of us have learned that treatment is most effective when we do everything perfectly. This occurs when the reinforcement schedule is exactly right, when we provide models and fade them at just the right time, when we choose stimuli for practice that contain only selected phonemic sequences, etc. We are not disappointed when change does not follow immediately; rather, we keep experimenting with our interventions and responses to the client. Further, we think of a sequence of treatment; no one expects the problem to be corrected in one session. When working with families it seems easy to forget this. Rather than viewing efforts to identify and use family resources over time, it is easy to become impatient and think of the family as being difficult rather than examining our own interventions and responses to families and viewing family participation as a process.

Families will not do everything perfectly in the beginning, if ever. However, by combining our expertise with theirs, we believe that our services often can be substantially more effective than if we worked alone with the client. Even if we *could* do treatment perfectly (and most of us can't), enlisting the family augments all treatment goals.

Empower Family Members

Family members cooperate most when the clinician is genuinely willing to empower them to change their own member's behavior and allows them to experience the satisfaction of improvement. When we work with individuals, we are accustomed to receiving a measure of credit for the change that we presumably evoked. When families are participants in treatment, the credit for change is shared with family members. In some cases, families may even attribute the change to a third factor or indicate that they do not know why the problem no longer exists.

Robert's parents, for example, attributed the fact that he no longer stuttered to their reducing the amount of sugar he was allowed to add to his breakfast cereal. This change was made along with rather far-reaching changes in their family interactive patterns, particularly with Robert. While our view of the relative importance of these two "causes" of change was different from that of the family's, the family made *both* changes. The important point is to reward parents for their involvement and empower them to continue to influence behavior rather than to quibble over reasons for change.

Appreciate Interactive Uniqueness

Families cooperate most when the clinician tries to understand the problem as it occurs in the interactive context of each family. Communicative disorders manifest themselves in different ways in different settings. For example, a child with a language delay, is likely to use more words at home with his/her family than at a preschool or in the presence of the clinician when the attention of everyone in the room is on the child. If families are to make interventions in the environment of the home, it is important that clinicians understand the manner in which family members experience the problem. As we begin to understand the problem within the context of the family then we may make valid and useful suggestions for them to carry out and build upon between sessions.

Create Idiosyncratic Assignments

Families cooperate most when the clinician understands each speech-language problem from the family's perspective and uses this information to give appropriate assignments that fit the family's understanding of the problem. Family members must understand the purpose and desired outcome of each assignment or they will be unable to accommodate to variations in the behavior and responses of their family member with a communicative disorder. When including families it may be a greater priority for the clinician to understand the problem from the point of view of the family than for the family to understand the problem from the clinician's perspective; both, however, are important.

CHAPTER 3

CONVENING THE FAMILY

On rare occasions, family members will request permission to participate in treatment. In these cases the clinician needs only to arrange a convenient time and place for the first meeting. More often, family members are not accustomed to being included in the speech-language-hearing treatment process, and it is unlikely that they will request involvement. The clinician must take the initiative if family participation is desired.

ASSESSING THE PROFESSIONAL CONTEXT

Many clinicians work in settings where parent conferences are an expected part of their services. These conferences can be used in a creative way to involve those families that the clinician believes can be helpful in treatment. Other clinicians may be able to utilize family visits to long-term or short-term rehabilitation facilities in a manner that uses the Family Based Treatment approach. Still others may use the private practice or clinic setting to develop their systemic treatment ideas. The clinician must evaluate possibilities for family involvement relative to the demands and expectations inherent in the professional context in which services will be offered.

Our work with families takes place in a university speech and hearing clinic, but the model is not limited to that context. When a clinician decides to become systemic in his/her approach to treatment, the next step is to define the system and choose a convening strategy that is likely to be successful.

DEFINING THE SYSTEM

After the clinician has decided to integrate family involvement into his/her professional setting, the clinician must determine whom to convene for the first meeting. We invite all of the family members who are significantly involved with the client. When the client is a child or adolescent living with both parents, we invite the parents as well as the child's siblings. If the child lives with one parent and the other parent is nearby, we also invite that person if the custodial parent is amenable to the idea. If mother or father has remarried or is closely involved with another person, the stepparent or friend is also invited to the family meeting.

Sometimes grandparents, aunts, uncles, cousins, and/or close family friends have daily, significant contact with our clients. These people are invited to the first session if the adult in charge thinks that this is a good idea. More often, extended family members are not invited to first sessions but are included in future sessions. This occurs when family members decide that extended family involvement will enrich the understanding and treatment of the communicative problem. We have been pleasantly surprised on several occasions to find grandparents, great-grandparents, aunts, cousins, playmates, baby-sitters and/or friends waiting with our families to join us in the treatment sessions. Some families know without being told that these important people are significant members of the client's communicative environment.

When the client is an adult, with that person's agreement we convene the spouse and any adult children who, with their spouses and children, are available to help in the treatment process. If the adult client lives alone or with one or both parents, the parents and/or available siblings are invited.

Occasionally the concept of family must be broadened

to include foster parents, child care workers, residential facility counselors, inpatient treatment personnel or other professionals who interact on a daily basis with clients. The convening goal is to invite family members and significant others based on their involvement with the client rather than beginning with a predetermined idea of a particular family organization. Families in our contemporary society are structured in a variety of ways. Therefore, the clinician must explore with the contact person all of the available options. The clinician should convene the people who are likely to expand an understanding of the interactive patterns in which the communicative disorder is embedded. All family members may not attend every session (if more than one meeting is desired), but when convened for the first meeting these people enrich the resource options available to the clinician and family.

The Telephone Call

Initial family contact is usually made by telephone. Sometimes an introductory letter precedes the phone call or, as occasionally has been the case for us, the clients must be contacted by letter because they have no telephone. In other cases, family visits to rehabilitation facilities generate a convening conversation. Often, however, telephone contact is the most efficient way to begin the convening process.

The joining process begins with the first interaction. Information is exchanged and the stage is set for family cooperation. For these reasons the clinician, rather than an appointment secretary, should make the initial contact. Following is an example of a convening telephone call as it might occur in our practice:

Mother: Hello
Clinician: Hello, this is Jim Andrews from the Speech & Hearing Clinic at Northern Illinois University. You called last week to arrange therapy for Johnny and I'm calling now to set that up.
Mother: Oh, good. I've been anxious to get him

	started.
Clinician:	It sounds like you're eager to get going; that's good. Let me tell you how I like to arrange the first session.
Mother:	OK
Clinician:	When I'm working with a child I like to have the important members of the family participate too. How does that sound to you?
Mother:	OK, I guess. I don't know if my husband can come though. He usually works late and isn't too involved with things like this.
Clinician:	He may not want to be very active in this, but it helps me a lot to get both parents' views of the problem when we get started. How about if we find a time that fits both of your schedules?
Mother:	It'll have to be in the evening. Do you want his brother and sister to come too?
Clinician:	Yes, everybody. Very young children don't have to come to every session but I like for everyone to attend the first one. Evening is fine. I can meet with you on Monday or Wednesday evening. Is 6:00 too early?
Mother:	Six would be fine on Wednesday. That will give us time to eat something and still not be too late for the kids.
Clinician:	Good. How old are your other children?
Mother:	Well, Christy, Johnny's sister, is eight and the baby, Paul, is 13 months.
Clinician:	I know it'll be a real effort for you to bring the whole family, but it helps me a lot to get both your ideas as well as your husband's about what might need to change. Also, it's helpful to see how Johnny communicates with his sister and baby brother.
Mother:	OK, actually I kind of like the idea of bringing everyone because Christy, especially, is better at understanding Johnny than any of

the rest of us.

Clinician: That's quite often the case. Brothers and sisters can be very helpful.

Mother: Well, let me talk to John (husband) and see if 6:00 on Wednesday is alright with him. (Leaves phone to discuss this with John — returns) He says it's OK, but doesn't think he can be much help.

Clinician: That's alright. Please tell him I really appreciate his taking the time to do this.

Mother: Is there anything we should do ahead of time?

Clinician: Well, yes. How about paying attention to the times when you and other family members can understand Johnny the best. This may not happen much before we meet, but if it does, please make note of it.

Mother: OK, I'll try, and we'll all be there on Wednesday at 6:00.

Clinician: Fine. The Clinic secretary will mail you a letter confirming the appointment and a map showing where you can park.

Several issues are raised in this convening conversation. The first is the role of Johnny's father. Most fathers do not expect to be involved in treatment services and most clinicians assume that the mother and child will be the treatment dyad if any family members participate. When the clinician adopts a systemic perspective, he/she knows that a clear understanding of family views and interactions will be elicited if, in a two parent family, father is included as well as mother. Furthermore, the concerns that parents share when a child has special needs are more easily addressed when both parents cooperate in the treatment process. Fathers are not always completely comfortable when they are first convened, but as their views are heard and respected and as their resources are used they usually join with their wives in working for speech-language change.

The second issue relates to the language used by the

convening clinician. Notice the frequent use of the phrase, "I need your help." We have found this to be the single most useful phrase in our convening practice. We believe that family members have information to offer that will make our clinical work more successful. Eight years of working with families has not changed our perspective on this issue.

Third, the clinician acknowledged the hassle involved in gathering family members together. This conveys empathy for the sometimes overwhelming burdens that accompany issues of disability.

Finally, an intervention has already taken place - even before the meeting occurs. Since Johnny's mother asked for a task, she was given one that will provide a beginning focus for the first interview.

Each convening conversation is idiosyncratic to the clinician/client/family situation. The following issues should be kept in mind:

1. Begin with the goal of convening all of the members of the household that are an immediate part of the client's communicative context.
2. Use language of cooperation and joining. Convey to family members at the outset that you know they will have valuable contributions to make to the treatment process.
3. Adopt an "experimental" attitude. Tell family members that this is a new idea - that it's a different way of working but that exciting things happen when we all work together.
4. Be persistent. Your friendly insistence that you need the family members' ideas may not be fully heard at first. As you persist in letting the contact person know the importance of family participation, this desire will be heard and acknowledged.

Scheduling

The desire to involve the members of the family creates complex scheduling issues. Some families can easily meet during regular daytime hours. Others can only meet after work and must be scheduled during the late afternoon and early evening. Flexibility in scheduling is critical to enlisting the cooperation of family members whose work hours vary.

The clinician, however, must also assure that his/her own busy schedule is accommodated so that resentment of giving up valuable personal time does not become an issue. It is best to work with only one family if this is all that can be reasonably done. The clinician must feel energized and challenged by the exciting issues associated with family treatment or the work will not be successful.

SUMMARY

Upon deciding to take a systemic approach and include families in the treatment process, the next task is to determine how best to convene families. Using language that signals participation and non-judgmental acceptance is an important ingredient when making the initial contact with a family member. All family members should be present for the clinician to view family interactions in which the disorder is embedded. A certain amount of friendly persistence may be necessary to achieve the goal of all family members being present. Flexibility in scheduling is necessary, but the clinician must arrange his/her time in a manner that makes working with families exciting and challenging if the approach is to be successful.

CHAPTER 4

SHARING AN UNDERSTANDING OF THE PROBLEM

There are many different ways of thinking about and understanding a communicative disorder. Just as the clinician shares a view of the problem when offering services based on the individual direct services model, it is important when working systemically for the clinician to develop and share a clear view of the problem. In many cases that view will be the one adopted by the family. On the other hand, unlike the individual model of services in which the different views held by family members may be irrelevant, when family members are participants in treatment, it is important for the clinician to understand their perspectives of the problem. The process in which each member of the family describes how the problem is experienced and understood is itself an intervention. That process usually leads the family to a greater understanding of the communicative disorder, the ways that family members have reacted to it, and interventions that each person has attempted. In turn, by learning this information the clinician is in a better position to understand solutions offered by the family. The clinician can then describe his/her own view of the problem in a way that is meaningful to the family and suggest solutions that accommodate the family's perspective.

When solutions suggested by the clinician are framed in language that fits the family's explanation and understanding of the problem, the suggestions may be said to be isomorphic to the family's view. Isomorphism is defined by

Hofstadter (1979) as a situation in which "two complex structures can be mapped onto each other, in such a way that to each part of one structure there is a corresponding part in the other structure" (p. 49). It is a family therapy principle that isomorphic assignments are more likely to be followed by families than assignments that do not relate to the family's understanding of the problem (deShazer, 1982). In other words, when the clinician understands the manner in which family members view the problem, he/she is in a position to offer more effective suggestions for change than if the family's views remain unknown. This and other features of assignments will be discussed in Chapter 6.

Since most speech-language pathologists employ a direct services model of clinical practice, traditionally we have assumed that the clinician should learn about the problem in order to personally treat it. On the other hand, when adopting a systemic perspective, the clinician's goal is to learn about the problem in a way that will permit everyone within the defined system to participate in treating it. This difference is substantial and affects all phases of the assessment process.

A number of counseling techniques may be used when interacting with family members. These enable the clinician to gain admittance to the family system, learn about the problem from the family, respond to their concerns, and enlist family members' participation in treatment. These are mentioned in conjunction with the process step of sharing an understanding of the problem described in this chapter, but will be discussed in Chapter 9. They include joining, clarifying, reflecting, summarizing, tracking interactive patterns, neutral questioning, and creative strategizing.

LEARNING THE FAMILY'S VIEW

Once the family is convened it is useful to begin the meeting with a few joining remarks. Reiterating that family members' willingness to participate is appreciated and explaining, again, why the entire family is involved is usually helpful since it is different than what they might have expected. Reminding the family that they are experts about their member, that they know more about their family member than anyone else, and that their help is needed to solve the problem assures them that they will be an integral part of the treatment team.

If children are involved it is helpful for parents to know the ground rules. When toys are set out the clinician may indicate that, if the parents wish, it is alright for the children to play with them. If there are objects that children should not disturb, this too should be indicated to the parents. This affirms at the outset the appropriate role of parents and indicates to them that they will be in charge of their children. The clinician may ask the family to bring a few toys and/or books that their child enjoys. This provides an even greater opportunity to learn about the family since it increases their control over the situation and tends to evoke their typical interactive style.

Very early it is likely that the clinician will notice behaviors and interactions that seem to be potential resources for intervention. These should be remembered for future use. It is not, however, inappropriate to comment upon something that a family member does that is exceptionally good. When a family member interacts with the client in such a way that the client responds with behavior that is obviously desirable, the clinician may speak positively of the intervention by talking about how well or how appropriately the client responded to that family member.

After addressing or attending to each family member, it is time to learn about the problem in a more formal manner. The clinician can begin this phase with a general statement such as, "Tell us how you experience_____'s speech-language problem." The family spokesperson usually responds first. Each person should be asked to respond and it is important to obtain each family member's view. After the family spokesperson has described the communicative problem from his/her perspective, a convenient method for making the transition to other family members is to say something like, "What do you think about that dad/mom? Do you agree with _____?" Children should also be offered the opportunity to respond if they have been listening to the conversation. The question to children may be addressed in the form of whether or not the brother or sister with the communicative disorder talks to them or whether or not they can understand their sibling. A request for a brief description of how they play together or, what the sibling does when the brother or sister cannot be understood may be made.

When the client is an adolescent or adult the same process is followed, but more attention is given to that person's view of the problem than is usually the case with young children. As the adolescent or adult expresses his/her views, the clinician must be careful to attend in a way that respects and acknowledges the client's hierarchical position in the family. As a general rule, attention to the views of the client increases with the individual's age until adulthood is reached.

Identifying Interactive Patterns

As family members are describing the problem, the clinician should attend to interactive patterns related to the communicative disorder. Tracking interactive sequences is a counseling technique that is used to learn about patterns in which the communicative problem is embedded. This technique leads to detailed descriptions of family interactions. Descriptive sequences of who says what and when can be developed, much like the script of a play. Each sequence in the script usually begins either with the client attempting to communicate or with a family member attempting to elicit responses or communication. From that point on, the clinician may ask about each behavioral event in the communicative sequence. He/she listens particularly for successful interactions (eg., where a parent helped the child, the child said the word, the intent of the child was understood, etc.) and also for those interactions which lead to frustration. Leading families to describe their communicative attempts at home and to think about things that they have done to help their family member usually results in a new level of understanding from which new insights are gained. Thus, it is most important at

this time not to give advice, but rather to listen and to use tracking and other techniques in order to gain a clear understanding of the problem as it occurs in the family environment.
Interactive sequences are likely to be acted out by family members during this first and subsequent sessions. As stated earlier, it is not too early for the clinician to compliment parents or other family members for those things that they say or do that appear to be helpful and which may facilitate change. We believe that it is far more useful to reinforce helpful things that family members say and do than to point out interactions that seem inappropriate. The latter are remembered, however, and discussed at later sessions if they continue to perpetuate the problem in a significant way.

It is particularly important, but sometimes difficult, to allow the family to show its interactive style. It is impossible to give meaningful assignments to families without knowing something about the environment in which they will be carried out. Allowing the family to "show itself" may at first seem like wasting time or losing control since, traditionally, we are accustomed to structuring the environment and reducing distractions to a minimum. However, a clinician gains insights and understands the problem more completely by observing and experiencing the environment in which the communicative disorder is manifested on an everyday basis. Further, the clinician is likely to personally sense the same feelings as the family as he/she joins the family system. We continue to be surprised by the power and ability of families to transmit to us their tension, frustration, sense of hopelessness, happiness, and other emotions.

Identifying Mobilization Points

If family members do not volunteer ways that they try to help their family member, we always ask. We listen for successful techniques to build upon and for unsuccessful techniques to avoid. From the family's point of view those strategies that seem to be successful, already make sense.

These will be easier for them to expand upon than new techniques which they have never used or experienced. We think of these successful, natural interactive techniques as mobilization points (Scott, 1984). They are one part of the family's resources and are excellent points from which to begin treatment. It is also useful to learn about typical family activities in which the client is involved, especially everyday events and times when one or more family members interact with the individual. These provide opportunities for family members to intervene. Learning about the client's favorite activities and typical daily events often suggests related opportunities for functional interventions by persons in the environment.

Listening for Agreement/Disagreement

During this initial portion of the interview and throughout the treatment process, it is important to listen for and talk about disagreements expressed between family members. Often, for example, one parent is more concerned about the perceived problem than the other. When this is the case and after talking openly about the two different views, we typically summarize the two perspectives and try to find a point of accommodation: "Dad, it sounds like you aren't really too concerned because you were also late in talking and Kathy may outgrow this just like you did. But, mom you're pretty worried about Kathy and would like to do something about it right now. Dad, would you be willing to participate in services to help ease your wife's concern?" In essentially every case in which this particular situation has come up, the answer to our question has been a genuine "yes." This intervention frees both parents to later observe and listen to the speech-language pathologist in a different way than if the issue had never been resolved. Both family members in this example become joined with one another and with the clinician in the effort to determine an appropriate level of service. We believe that disagreements which are ignored will return to impede progress. It is very important, then, to listen carefully for these, talk about them, and try to find a point of accommodation. This is not to imply that family members all experience the communicative disorder in the same way or that each should think about it like everyone else in the family. These disagreements should be highlighted, but no point of agreement will be sought. Rather, the clinician will determine interventions that take advantage of the different experiences and perspectives. It is helpful to talk about differences positively. For example, "Brian is lucky to have both of your influences. Dad, you like to roughhouse with him and don't worry about how much he talks; on the other hand, mom, you're concerned about how he'll fit into school next year and you like to stimulate him academically. Both of these are important." Assignments that follow should capitalize on the two different parental styles.

A frequent question which arises is whether the person with the communicative disorder should be present during this portion of the interview. Without that individual present, it is impossible to assess his/her role as a communicator in the family system, the manner in which family members interact with that person, and the communicative environment of the family. These interactions are so important that they should be observed even if detailed questions about the individual with the handicap are not asked in his/her presence. In all but a very small number of cases we have included the family member with the problem in the room with everyone else. That person nearly always knows that he/she is the reason for the conference. Further, the conversation about the problem is conducted in a caring manner. This may be quite different from the manner in which the problem has been discussed at home and also different from the giving of advice or cajoling that may have occurred in other contexts. On the other hand, if it seems inappropriate to talk about the problem in the client's presence, don't do it. A clinician's judgment should never be superseded by the dictates of a particular approach.

DEVELOPING THE CLINICIAN'S VIEW

After learning about the problem from the family's perspective, observing interactions in which the problem is embedded, and observing the manner in which the client communicates, a more detailed assessment is necessary. At this point, the clinician needs to learn more about the problem, and to determine additional information about possibilities for change. Since the bulk of change is likely to occur in interactions with family members, it is important to include the family as active participants in the assessment. This not only leads to further information about the communicative disorder, but allows the clinician to determine the nature of family resources that are available.

Family Participation

The specific manner in which the family participates in the assessment varies with the type of communicative disorder. A primary goal, however, is to include family members in such a way that they appreciate the problem more completely and see themselves as capable of eliciting change in their own family member. The latter is a source of empowerment for families. It usually is very rewarding to families to be able to change even a small aspect of their family member's communicative ability very early in the treatment process.

The clinician may begin by attending to that part of the problem that concerns family members most. For example, when the primary concern is articulation, administration of an articulation test can yield useful information about family resources for participating in treatment. The clinician can start by briefly explaining the nature of the test and asking a family member to administer it. Seating is rearranged to allow family members and the clinician to sit close to the child. Initially, as each picture is named, the clinician may comment on the child's accuracy of production usually adding a brief statement about how the particular sound is produced. When a sound is misarticulated, the clinician provides a model for the child and elicits imitation. Appropriate feedback is given to the child by the clinician. Family members observe these interactions and after the clinician has done this two or three times, the member administering the test is asked to do the stimulability testing/trial therapy. From that point, the clinician attends to both the parent and the child and comments upon the performance of each. Just as verbal directions and reinforcement are traditionally used to shape the behavior of clients, the same techniques are used with the family member. The reactions of other family members are also observed and the ability of the parent administering the test is positively described to them. It is particularly useful to comment on the helpful techniques that the family member is using. For example, "You let him know really well that you were pleased when he corrected the way he made that sound" or "I like the way you're exaggerating the sound to help her; that calls it to her attention." Just as we want individual clients to feel good about their ability to change, we want parents and other family members to have that same sense of satisfaction. The clinician may then reinforce both the parent and the child, but gradually the role of reinforcing the child is turned over to the parent. The clinician is commenting throughout on the child's speech, teaching the family as the clinician learns. The clinician may also compare performance on the test to spontaneous speech as heard earlier by the clinician or commented upon by family members.

When the problem is language delay with a young child, the clinician can begin the clinical assessment by asking an appropriate family member to play with the child for a few minutes. During this time, the clinician may observe features such as ability to obtain a shared focus of attention with the child; the extent to which the parent follows the child's lead, provides models, and otherwise stimulates the child; the frequency with which the parent reinforces desired behavior, etc. Both the child's responses and the adult's style of interaction are observed and mentally compared with earlier descriptions and observations. Gradually, the clinician inserts himself/herself into the activity. Often the first step is to comment on either something the parent is doing well or to join the parent in his/her frustration by commenting upon something that is difficult (eg., getting the child's attention). Rather than "taking over," the clinician should *join* the parent(s) and child in play. While interacting with the child, the clinician can comment on the child's responses to interventions and playing style. This interaction permits the clinician to determine the client's responses to different forms of stimulation and reward and to gain a sense of those behaviors that will be easiest to change. Gradually, the clinician may suggest a new activity to experiment further if the parents or the child do not change activities on their own.

When the client is older, the interactive context for this portion of the evaluation is usually more conversational. For example, the family with an aphasic or head-injured member may be asked to engage in conversation to demonstrate some of the features that they described earlier during the interview. In this case the clinician observes the interactions and may begin to make comments, particularly noting helpful interventions made by family members. In some cases, of course, these involve a passive behavior such as waiting; whereas in others, the interaction may be more active such as saying the first sound of a word. We especially want to notice the reaction of the client to these attempts to help. If the intervention made communication easier, this should be confirmed with the client, if possible, and with the family members. Such behavior may be a mobilization point. If the client appeared to become angry or frustrated by the intervention, this too should be discussed. These brief discussions often lead to descriptions of related attempts to help and the effectiveness of these efforts. These, too, may be demonstrated by the family during the session.

Gradually, the clinician becomes part of the conversation and makes his/her own interventions. Since these are done with the family present as participants, they will observe the effectiveness of the clinician's suggestions and comment upon how they relate to techniques they have tried. In the case of a head-injured mildly apraxic teenager, for example, we suggested that he emphasize the rhythm of his speech. At the first session we selected phrases we heard him use spontaneously in interactions with his parents and siblings. By having him practice these we were able to develop an assignment at the first meeting that everyone understood. Since the young man enjoyed playing the drums, his mother suggested that he tap out the rhythm of selected words, phrases, and sentences on his leg. His older brother suggested phrases that the client tended to use in conversation while his father told us the words that were especially difficult for his son to say. The teenager also contributed to this discussion and made suggestions. Through the combined efforts of the clinician and the family, an evaluation of functional communication took place, goals were set, and an assignment for the first week was developed.

Standardized Testing

When using a systemic approach, the clinician may increasingly evaluate communication in functional contexts and rely less and less on standardized tests. While the former leads directly to interventions (as described above), the latter usually does not. When a standardized test is administered, however, one can begin by explaining the purpose and nature of the test. The clinician can explain that the client may not respond to some items that family members are sure he/she knows. Other responses, however, may be pleasantly surprising to the family. The clinician should make it clear that the test must be administered in a particular manner. The family may be advised that the group will discuss the client's performance after the test is completed. Further, the clinician may add that he/she realizes that it is sometimes difficult to watch quietly as a test is administered. Nevertheless, the family should watch. However, if the family includes small children who may distract the client it is appropriate to have someone take the children to another room while the test is being administered. After completing the test, families usually want to talk about their observations and compare them with their everyday experience. Sometimes, as a result of watching, families will come to a new realization of the seriousness and severity of the problem. In this case, the clinician can follow the family's lead and discuss the problem in more detail. Counseling skills are used to respond to emotional statements and behavior. When families are expressing their concern and/or grief, it is no time for advice, suggestions, cheering up, or minimizing the problem. The most helpful thing that the clinician can do at that time is to respond to the feelings being expressed.

SUMMARY

In the first phase of the assessment we are suggesting that the clinician learn each family member's view of the problem and listen particularly for (1) interactive sequences in which the problem is embedded; (2) mobilization points; (3) times when family members come together with the communicatively handicapped member; (4) activities which both the handicapped member and other family members enjoy doing together; and (5) agreement/disagreement between family members. This information may be enhanced by observing interactions as they are acted out during the session.

After learning about the family's view of the problem, the clinical evaluation is performed with family participation. It is suggested that the clinician talk about what he/she is learning throughout this portion of the assessment so that by the time it is completed the family will have learned about the problem along with the clinician. This allows the family to participate more effectively in treatment than if the clinician were to conduct the evaluation privately.

CHAPTER 5

AGREEING ON CHANGES AND SETTING GOALS

Both the speech-language pathologist and the family will be burgeoning with new information after sharing an understanding of the problem. For the family, the process has involved hearing one another's view of the problem often for the first time. They will have discovered points of agreement and disagreement and outlined the specifics of their interactions with the family member having a communicative disorder. Having heard one another describe what each person has done to help, the family is likely to be thinking about the problem and potential solutions in a new and different way. The speech-language pathologist's professional energy has been focused on learning about the problem from the different family members including the family member with the communicative disorder. The clinician has observed enactments of interactive patterns, conducted a clinical assessment, and developed a view of the problem. Finally, the clinician has been thinking about how his/her professional knowledge can be linked to the family's resources. Both family members and the clinician have a developing sense of the problem and of the early possibilities for change. The outcome now depends upon the clinician's expertise in applying his/her knowledge in a manner that will be useful to the family. The skill required is quite different than that which would be used in a direct service delivery model. It is natural to have reservations about one's ability to do this; sometimes mistakes will be made just as errors are made in individual treatment sessions. The difference, however, is that no one knows about mistakes of judgment made in a closed client-clinician dyad. Working with families requires both confidence in one's clinical ability and an open style of interacting.

When the first step of treatment is not obvious and clear to everyone, the clinician can begin this goal-setting phase of services by asking the family to suggest one or two behaviors in which even a small change would be significant to them. If their request is not inconsistent with the principles of good speech-language pathology practice, it should be honored. In fact, rather than refusing an inappropriate request, the clinician can suggest modifications to make the request an appropriate goal. More often, families prefer that the professional decide what the goals should be. By this time in the process, families have been involved in a mutual sharing of ideas and information and understand that they will be active participants in making changes. As respect is shown for the family they, in turn, become respectful of the opinions of the speech-language pathologist in a manner characteristic of "equal partners." Even when the clinician sets the treatment goals, he/she can offer the family an opportunity to confirm or ratify the decision. This is an important step since it is critical that family members understand and agree to the specifics of the particular behavior to be changed. Also, it confirms the hierarchical structure of family, client, and clinician and expands the joining process by showing respect for the family's opinion. This procedure should be followed throughout the treatment process.

Resources of the family, including mobilization points, form a major basis for setting goals and determining behaviors to be changed. The process of family participation in changing the behavior of one of its members early in treatment is probably as important as the details of the behavior selected and the magnitude of change relative to the overall problem. Just as we design goals and procedures in a direct services model so that the individual will be highly successful, in a systemic model the clinician will want to arrange

Agreeing on Changes and Setting Goals

success for both the client and the family members participating in treatment. The clinician's internal process of connecting his/her expertise with the family's idiosyncratic style is called *creative strategizing*. The clinician attempts to combine all of the information he/she has learned about the family's view of the problem, the family style and structure, mobilization points, and the clinician's own view of what can and should be changed in order to develop appropriate goals and related assignments. This process is repeated at subsequent sessions, but additional information is added based upon the outcome of assignments.

Three examples of first session information follow. The initial goal(s) and assignments that were developed with these families are also described. These case studies serve to describe the process more than to exemplify perfection!

FAMILY NUMBER ONE

Present at the first session: Kate, 4 years, 2 months; mother, Mildred; live-in boy friend, Jerry; and, eight year old brother, Greg. Mother is divorced.

Chief Complaint: Difficulty understanding Kate's speech.

Family Characteristics and Interactions:
1. Kate talks > mother can't understand what Kate says > mother asks Kate to repeat what she said > (a) Kate speaks more clearly > (mother rewards Kate, sometimes) > mother responds, or (b) mother still can't understand Kate and tells Kate this > Kate walks away.
2. Kate has opportunities to talk; family members wait for her and try to understand what she says.
3. Mother and friend are capably in charge of the children and have established a calm pleasant environment.

Mobilization Points:
1. Mother reinforces Kate and Kate responds well to her praise.
2. Mother's friend enjoys singing songs, reading books to the children, and making up stories with the children.
3. Kate corrects many of her error sounds with minimal stimulation.

Speech-Language Characteristics:
1. Simplification of blends
2. t/k prevocalically
3. w/l or /l/ omitted
4. Inconsistent errors on multisyllabic words with moderate difficulty sequencing syllables
5. Inconsistent use of /f/ for plosives and fricatives in blends (eg., tr > fr; gr > fr; dr > fr; gl > fr; br > fr; kr > fr)
6. Inconsistent use of me/I

Initial Goals:
1. Correct use of /k/ in prevocalic position
2. Improve ability to sequence sounds and syllables accurately by attending to the rhythm of speech

First Assignment:
1. Make a list of songs you like to sing with Kate and bring it next week. When you sing with her this week, listen especially for three syllable words in the songs and notice how they sound.
2. Find excuses for Kate to hear you say a lot of words that start with the "k" sound (eg., when playing, singing, telling stories, etc.). Emphasize them a little by pausing briefly and saying them just a little louder than usual.

After discussing the assignment with the family and demonstrating the technique, the family spontaneously named some words beginning with the /k/ sound that came up frequently in conversations with Kate. These were: comb, car, Kate, come, curtain, and kitchen. A session was scheduled for the next week.

In a one hour session, a good deal was learned about Kate's speech and how her family could help her. More information would be developed in the continuing weeks, but enough was learned at the first session to establish initial goals and procedures to elicit change. The resources of the mother became especially apparent when she administered an articulation test. She learned immediately how to stimulate and reward Kate in a kind, patient, natural manner. Kate's brother helped us learn about Jerry's' story-telling assets and enjoyment of play when we asked about times that the family came together. It was clear from the beginning that the adults were in charge of the children and that family members' rights were important and protected. As we joined the family system we sensed a combination of respect, enjoyment, and playfulness.

The goals were selected by us, but the family was given the opportunity to agree or disagree with them. The /k/ was selected as a target sound since Kate used it correctly in many phonetic contexts and her mother was able to stimulate a correct production rather easily. Further, both adults were able to identify it and easily distinguish it from /t/. Note, however, that their initial assignment was not to correct Kate's production, but rather to let her hear the sound. Interestingly, while playing alone at the next session, Kate used the sound correctly in words she said aloud, as the adults were discussing the success of the assignment. Emphasizing Kate's use of rhythm, we believed, would provide a framework for the general improvement of articulation. This goal was particularly directed toward improving her inconsistent sequential errors in multisyllabic words. The family's enjoyment of singing songs with Kate provided a vehicle for a beginning emphasis upon the rhythm of speech.

During the first session, the family's resources were called to their attention prior to giving the assignment. Reinforcing a family's resources has the effect of enlisting their cooperation and strengthening family members' abilities and confidence to change their own member's behavior.

Setting goals and determining methods for changing behavior so that these may be utilized has the effect of enabling families to participate effectively.

FAMILY NUMBER TWO

Present at the first session: Steve, 16 years and recently head injured; mother, Margaret; father, John; sister, Karen, 19 years; brother, Ed, 14 years.

Chief Complaint: Slurred hesitant speech and difficulty finding words following a head trauma.

Family Characteristics and Interactions:
1. The family is appropriately attentive to Steve and wants to help him. Their main concern has been his health and survival, but they are now eager to normalize his life.
2. Steve's mother and sister do most of the talking for the family, but defer appropriately to Steve and allow him to speak for himself.
3. Steve is given time to think of words and has ample opportunities to participate in conversation

Mobilization Points:
1. Steve has figured out that his speech is best when he speaks slowly and deliberately. He tries to help himself in this way.
2. Steve's parents have encouraged his musical and theatrical interests through private lessons in both areas. Further, he has been active in athletics and is a good student.
3. The entire family is interested in music; both parents work professionally in that area.
4. Steve and his family brought a list of words that were particularly difficult for him to say.

Speech-Language Characteristics:
1. Mild verbal apraxia
2. Mild word finding problem

3. Sentence formulation and grammatical structure were very good
4. Speech less animated, less colloquial, and more monotonous in pitch and loudness than prior to the injury. Steve's friends described him as "more formal" and "not as fun loving" as previously.
5. Very mild dysarthria associated with weakness on the right side of the lips and tongue. Tongue deviated to the right upon protrusion. No apparent atrophy or fasciculations.
6. Immediate memory mildly impaired.

Initial Goal:
To reduce the apraxic-related errors in conversation

First Assignment:
1. Experiment with directing speech movements with your head or tapping with your hand to exaggerate and get a sense of the rhythm of speech.
2. Have "think rhythm" conversations with family members in which you exaggerate the rhythm of speech for a minute or two.
3. Practice the seven words that you brought which are especially difficult for you in the phrases below. Exaggerate the rhythm.
I'm going to be *practicing*
Tomorrow is *Thursday*
It's got the *same sound*
Don't be *gullible*
Don't be *facetious*
DeKalb, *Illinois*
Topics of *conversation*

The initial goal was related to one of the concerns expressed by Steve and his family. The intervention procedures grew out of a combination of Steve's discovery that he could improve his articulation if he spoke more deliberately, the clinician's knowledge of the nature of apraxia, and practice during the session in which Steve's articulation improved greatly when he exaggerated the rhythm of speech. His ability to sense the rhythm of speech was connected to the family's musical ability and interests and Steve's excellent pre-injury drum playing ability. This prompted the family to experiment with Steve in a different manner than if that association had not been made.

Steve was reinforced for his introspective ability to figure out that there were things he could do to help himself. The family's obvious concern for Steve and their desire to restore normalcy to his life were positively regarded by the clinician. Subsequent assignments capitalized on his voice lessons, acting interest, drumming ability, his pre-injury sense of humor, and his desire to succeed academically. The latter two became mobilization points as both behaviors began to improve.

FAMILY NUMBER THREE

Present at the first session: Sam, 3 years, 10 months; mother, Lana; father, Gene; brother, Tom, 18 months.

Chief Complaint: Parents can't understand Sam's speech.

Family Characteristics and Interactions:

1. Sam's mother is the family spokesperson and is worried about Sam's communicative performance. Sam's father is quiet, not very worried about Sam, but supportive of his wife.
2. Much of the family's interaction focuses upon or relates to Sam. Interactions are designed to promote his communicative attempts.
3. Tom plays by himself very well. His speech-language appear to be developing normally.
4. Sam and his parents look at books, play with picture cards, and listen to children's music and television shows together.
5. Sam's father plays "hop on pop" with Sam in which Sam climbs on his dad as dad lies on the floor.

Agreeing on Changes and Setting Goals

Mobilization Points:
1. Sam's mother is able to understand what Sam wants even if Sam doesn't use words to express himself.
2. Both parents enjoy playing with toys with Sam and use these times as opportunities to stimulate Sam's language.
3. Both parents use a technique in which they point to their mouths and say "tell me" when Sam doesn't use words to communicate. He sometimes responds by saying a word or two or by repeating "tell me" and then saying a word.
4. Sam imitates words over 50% of the time. His parents use this by asking a question, answering the question, and cheering for Sam when he imitates the word.
Parent: What's this Sam?
Parent: That's a car.
Sam: That car.
Parent: Good, Sam. That's a car, good for you! Yea!
5. When the parents don't know what Sam wants, they say "show me" and Sam sometimes points to the object.
6. Sam likes to sit by his mother as she looks at books and names the pictures for Sam.
7. The parents name things for Sam more than they ask him questions about the names of objects.

Speech-Language Characteristics:
1. Sam rarely spontaneously initiates verbal interaction in any form whether it be naming objects, pictures, or people; expressing a need; or greeting people. He says "no" in situations in which he is verbally stimulated, as if to mean "stop."
2. Sam communicates negation by saying "no."
3. We were unable to obtain reliable pointing responses to pictures or objects he named. The parents reported no better success.

4. It is difficult to achieve a shared focus of attention with Sam.
5. Sam attends to the details of toys (eg., the wheel of a toy tractor) and tends to "study" these rather than play with toys symbolically.
6. Sam did not interact visually with his parents during the session.

Initial Goal:
To develop nonverbal social interactions with Sam as a basis for communication.

First Assignment:
1. Notice the extent to which you are able to join Sam in a shared activity (eg., playing with toys) and the extent to which he will join you when you initiate the activity.
2. You do an excellent job of encouraging Sam to communicate. Keep doing these things.

In this case, there was an obvious discrepancy between the parents' stated view of the problem and our view. Although the parents framed the problem in terms of their ability to understand Sam's speech, their efforts to help him were nearly all designed to encourage language usage. This discrepancy was discussed and his parents agreed with our initial goal even though they were under the impression that the goal could be achieved quickly.

Because of the difference in opinions, a "noticing assignment" was given for the first week rather than an intervention type of assignment. However, the parents were complimented for the excellent techniques that they had developed to help Sam use language, and they were encouraged to continue those activities. They were instructed to bring one or two of Sam's books and some favorite toys to the next session, one week later, to demonstrate their observations about establishing a shared focus of attention with Sam.

SUMMARY

Perhaps the most challenging component of Family Based Treatment is linking the clinician's expertise with the resources and style of the family. It is at this point in the process that the clinician begins to truly empower families. Three examples are provided to illustrate the connection between family and speech-language characteristics and first assignments. The translation of data to appropriate goals is the result of creative strategizing. The degree of success of the process becomes evident at the next meeting with the family.

CHAPTER 6

ASSIGNMENTS

Each session culminates in an assignment based upon the professional judgment of the clinician. In the individual model, assignments are given to further the efforts of the clinician. These are often given without thought as to whether their purpose is understood by family members, whether they will fit the family's style of interaction, or whether or not they are based upon family resources. These are typically "sent home" with the client and usually involve some kind of intervention such as practicing a set of words or phrases with the client.

When families participate in treatment, assignments are given to help them promote change within the communicative interactions of the natural environment. Successful creative strategizing and a resulting appropriate assignment relies heavily upon the clinician's ability to listen and learn. The clinician must connect his/her understanding of the problem with that of the family's, and develop a treatment plan that capitalizes upon the resources of the family. This connection not only enlists but maintains family participation. As the family participates, they are often able to improve upon assignments and tailor them even more specifically to their own unique situation. Toward this end, we use three types of assignments.

THREE TYPES OF ASSIGNMENTS

Noticing Assignments

Sometimes the clinician may want family members to become more familiar with some of the details of their member's communicative handicap. In this case an assignment is given which leads the family to learn more about the problem. This is called a "noticing assignment" because it usually begins with a word or phrase such as "Notice" or "Pay attention to" some particular aspect of communication. For example, it may be that the clinician wants family members to attend to a particular aspect of the client's behavior or variations in that behavior. Some examples are: "Notice the way Mark uses past tense verbs and write down some examples."; "Pay attention to the situations in which Jack is most fluent and be ready to tell us about these next time we meet."; "Pay attention to the situations in which Janice talks the most and let us know next time what these are."; and "Notice how often and under what circumstances Colleen imitates words or sounds you say to her."

Another purpose of noticing assignments is to learn more about the behavior of parents, siblings, the client, spouses, or other family members. Often it is not only the clinician who learns from these, but family members as well. Both purposes are legitimate. A family can be more effective in carrying out direct interventions when they are familiar with the circumstances in which they will be asked to intervene. This type of assignment often leads to a greater appreciation of resources about which family members had been only generally aware or to the previously unnoticed effect of environmental variables. An example of an assignment like this is, "Notice Steve's successes in controlling or handling situations well." This assignment was given to the family of a young child who stuttered. They had just noticed that the child was maturing in a positive way and that fluency was improved when the child had some control over particular situations. Other examples are: "Pay attention to the 'pause time' after John finishes speaking and before someone else speaks";

"Notice how often you interact with Julie by asking a question or asking her to repeat something you have said"; and "Pay attention to what you do when Kate indicates that she wants something."

This noticing type of assignment is often given to family members to build upon something that they have brought up during the session. John's parents, in the above example, had noticed that John's stuttering seemed to be related to their rate of speech as well as to that of his older brother's. After discussing this and having them play with John while they attempted to slow their rate it became apparent that even when they slowed down they were all quick to talk the instant that John paused. The assignment was given in order to help them appreciate this aspect of speaking rate. As is often the case, the family not only noticed their conversational turn-taking behavior during the next week, but attempted to do something about it. Thus, a noticing assignment became an intervention assignment as the family developed a better understanding of factors related to their child's fluency. Such assignments frequently have the effect of changing the behavior of family members since their attention becomes focused on communication. The assignment to "notice" may also help family members gain a new appreciation for the positive aspects of their member's behavior or even an appreciation for positive things that they are already doing to help. When family members grow in appreciation of their own resources, they usually become even more effective participants in treatment.

The clinician's *intent* in developing and delivering an assignment is critical to the assignment's success. Giving a noticing assignment so that a family will discover how "bad" they are will not work! Rather, it will serve to alienate the family from the clinician and make the family less able to participate in treatment. The clinician's intent must be to be helpful and to nudge the therapeutic process forward rather than to demonstrate his/her superiority or to expose weaknesses of the family.

Another purpose of assigning a family a noticing assignment might be to help them or the clinician learn about the effect of the environment upon the individual's communicative disorder. For example, an assignment to notice whether Tim talked more when the television was off than on was given to one family. They had reported that their video cassette recorder was not working and they had noticed that Tim, who was four and talking very little, seemed to be interacting with them more when they were not watching so much TV. Admittedly, there is overlap among these examples of noticing assignments when one attempts to determine whether the assignment was given to describe the child's behavior, family member's behaviors, or the effect of the environment on communication. The examples may, however, serve to stimulate the reader's imagination and creativity in developing successful interventions of the noticing variety. In every case, the goal of an assignment should be to move toward speech-language change.

Intervention Assignments

A second type of assignment is more traditional and involves assigning family members something overt to do or something to refrain from doing. This type of assignment is called an "intervention assignment" since it involves an action. Intervention assignments are made to alter the communicative environment of the client in one of three ways: (1) by family members initiating interaction or responding to the client in a particular way; (2) by family members interacting among themselves in a particular manner; or (3) by family members engaging in some beneficial activity with the client. Some examples are as follows: "Use family photos to elicit past tense verbs and restate what Mark says using the correct form of the verb."; "Make a tape recording of some of your interactions with Michael in which you reward him and restate what he says."; "I think you're right that asking David to say words isn't working. This week, when you look at books, you name things and point to them. Go slowly and leave 'spaces' for him to talk if he wants to (eg., 'I see a ....car')."

In the above example in which the family was asked to make a tape recording of members interacting with Michael, one purpose was to give us a better idea of exactly how they were rewarding and restating Michael's utterances. The intent was to reward the things that they were doing well and thus encourage them. No one thought of the assignment in any other than a positive and helpful way. This is an important point because in some cases clinicians may tend to look for negative features about families rather than positive attributes. Families who have positive feelings about their ability to participate will increase in skill and effectiveness. Families who are made to feel inept and inadequate will respond by being exactly that.

It is important to make intervention assignments systemic, that is, something that one or more family members do within the context of natural interactions. This is as opposed to assigning practice or drills outside of natural interaction. The latter is typical of individual treatment. One should not attempt to duplicate the work that a speech-language pathologist would do by assigning those same tasks to family members. Rather, the clinician should attempt to maintain the advantage of the natural environment by assigning communication techniques and particular ways in which typical family interactions may be modified to help the client. Occasionally, however, this is not possible. When drill-work seems appropriate, the clinician may wish to change to an individual approach or to employ a combined family-individual approach in which family sessions are supplemented by one or more individual sessions per week. Even when a change is made to a direct intervention model, the clinician should maintain a family perspective. Further, having begun treatment with family participation, the family will remain active members of the team. The commitment must be to change and methods that will best effect change.

Assessing Effectiveness Assignments

A third type of assignment is given to assess the

results of particular interventions and of the overall treatment plan. These are called "assessing effectiveness" assignments. Some examples are as follows: "Listen to find out whether or not Mark spontaneously revises sentences to use the correct verb form."; "Julie is beginning to hold brief 'conversations' with you. Write down some examples of these in a script form."; and "Write down words that you hear Gretchen say spontaneously this week."

The clinician may compare the information derived from "assessing effectiveness" assignments to the behavior observed during the session. Family members can point out similarities to what they have heard at home or in some cases describe the differences between the client's home behavior and that elicited during the session. This provides additional data to be combined with other information gained during the session in order to develop the next assignment. The information may also be used to highlight the role and ability of family members to stimulate change in the client.

Assignments are the clinician's link to change. The success or failure of treatment hinges on the appropriateness of assignments and the manner in which assignments are delivered.

DELIVERING THE ASSIGNMENT

The single most important factor in delivering an assignment is the clinician's intent. The clinician who has a genuinely helpful intention for each assignment is unable to hide this from families. Similarly, families recognize the intentions of clinicians who give assignments designed to uncover the family's ineptness, incomplete knowledge, and/or inadequacy. The clinician with good intentions may give an inappropriate assignment but at worst, the family reports that they were unable to complete it. The clinician who highlights a family's negative features, is unlikely to learn the results of assignments since family members will probably react by withdrawing and devaluing their resources.

Second, it is usually most appropriate to deliver the

assignment by making reference to something that the family has already mentioned, something that has been previously discussed with the family, or something that occurred during the session that was pertinent. In other words, successful assignments are isomorphic to the family's view of reality. It is also helpful for families to view the assignment in context, that is as an integral part of the total treatment plan rather than as an isolated act. Appropriate assignments usually follow in such a tight, logical order that families are not usually surprised by the next step. However, it is helpful for the clinician to make this sequential connection when delivering the assignment.

Third, whenever possible, the clinician should give assignments in rewarding contexts. That is, the time of planning with the family is often a good time to evaluate their contribution to the progress that the family member is making. Because the clinician attempts to identify those things that family members do well, it is natural to reward the particular efforts of families in conjunction with delivering the next assignment. For example, "Allen is responding well to your efforts to say words to him rather than asking him to talk. I know it's difficult and you're doing a good job. This week, try pausing some of the time when you are looking at the book with him; say a partial sentence and pause. If he doesn't say the word, you go ahead and say it and go on. Keep up the good work of not asking him questions."

Fourth, the clinician should ask the family whether or not they think the assignment is possible to do and if they think it will be effective. Usually they will respond positively; sometimes, however, they have concerns about it. When this occurs, use listening skills to determine what is concerning them and modify the assignment or give a new one. It is very important that family members understand the assignment and believe that they will be able to carry it out.

Fifth, the clinician should demonstrate the assignment and then ask members of the family to try it. One demonstrates with the member having the communicative problem so that the family can see exactly what is being asked of them and see their member's response. This is followed by family members doing the assignment. The clinician can then compare the client's responses to the family with those elicited by the clinician. As might be expected, the client usually responds better to members of his/her family than to the clinician. This allows the clinician to emphasize the familial bond, thus again, reinforcing the family. As family members carry out the assignment, the clinician can also critically evaluate their performance and give them feedback. Reward those things that they do well and suggest modifications of behaviors that are significant but which could be improved. This is done as family members are carrying out the assignment so that they have the opportunity to try again immediately and to ask questions if the client seems not to be responsive.

Finally, after talking about the assignment the clinician should give it to the family in writing. The format for assignments includes the date, the names of those present, reinforcing remarks, the specific assignment(s), and the date/time of the next session.

SUMMARY

The activities of each session are directed toward the development and delivery of an assignment which will advance speech-language improvement in the family member with a communicative disorder. Most successful assignments are systemic in nature in that they are to be carried out during natural interactions. While attempts are made to match the assignment with the style of the family and take into account factors such as roles, rules, and hierarchy, families are expected to modify the assignment to make for a better "fit" as they carry out the activities. This is natural and possible when family members understand the purpose of the assignment and the goal toward which it is directed.

Three types of assignments are available to the clinician. One is a *noticing assignment,* given for family members to learn more about the problem, for the clinician to learn more about the family and/or the client, or to strengthen a new insight or perception that family members express. A second type of assignment is an *intervention assignment,* one in which family members are directed to do something or not to do something. Finally, an *assessing effectiveness assignment* is given to determine the effect of the treatment program or to call family members' attention to change that has occurred.

Assignments are most successful when they are delivered in the spirit of good intentions and when the clinician relates them to existing information with which the family is familiar. Further, assignments are most effective when they are explained in the context of reinforcement, when family members are invited to comment upon their appropriateness, and when they are demonstrated by the clinician and practiced by the family.

CHAPTER 7

ASSESSING TREATMENT EFFECTIVENESS

In the Family Based Treatment services model the most significant speech-language changes occur between sessions when the clinician is not with the family. While change is related to the events of the preceding session, including the assignment, it is usually difficult to assign a one-to-one causal relationship between the actions taken by the clinician and the results manifested by the client. This is because interactions are not subject to the same rules of reinforcement as simple actions (Keeney, 1983). When one works with individuals in the traditional direct services approach, much of the attention is directed toward stimulating and rewarding particular behaviors. Examples of these are the use of a specific grammatical construction such as past tense, accurate production of a particular phoneme, reading a sentence while maintaining a clear non-harsh voice, and voluntarily repeating the first syllable of a word and maintaining control. These behaviors may be referred to as "simple actions" and, conveniently, they are subject to the laws of reinforcement. They are the primary focus of most individual treatment sessions. The clinician manipulates a simple behavioral action during each treatment session and records the outcome or success rate.

ATTEND TO SIMPLE ACTIONS AND INTERACTIONS

Simple actions are also attended to in Family Based Treatment in that the clinician observes the manner in which different family members facilitate and elicit specific behaviors of the member having the speech-language problem. The clinician makes suggestions in that regard, and demonstrates the usefulness of reinforcement. In addition, however, there is attention to family interactive patterns since some of these may facilitate change while others may be perpetuating the problem. The use of counseling techniques such as tracking, listening, and clarifying, in and of themselves, sometimes alters the ways in which family members view the communicative disorder. This, in turn, results in modifications in communicative patterns and change in the member with the problem. The exact cause of speech-language change may be difficult to identify due to the complexity of systemic transformations. These transformations include new family interactions, perspectives, and relationships with the larger network of friends and relatives.

Rakeem, nearly three years old, was the first born son of Middle Eastern parents. He lived at home with his mother and father and his younger sister. Not only did Rakeem have very limited expressive language, but his sister was quickly "gaining on him" and was approaching Rakeem's level of performance and even surpassing him in terms of interactive use and spontaneity of language.

Rakeem's mother seemed to know instinctively many appropriate techniques for stimulating Rakeem's language development. An interactive pattern had developed, however, in which Rakeem's father showed disdain for Rakeem at a level which varied with the intensity of effort used by Rakeem's mother to help her son. She would, for example, play with Rakeem, direct her attention to objects in which he seemed interested, and name them. Her desire for Rakeem to imitate her was evident even though she frequently did not ask this of Rakeem. As Rakeem's mother attempted to facilitate language development, Rakeem's father showed disgust for Rakeem's lack of talking and made disparaging sounds and comments to his wife as she attempted to help Rakeem. This, in turn, caused her to try even harder to encourage Rakeem to imitate her. In addition, she responded by defending the child to his father by saying something to the effect that he *could* name the toys if he wanted to, that he was improving, that he was trying his best, etc. Father reacted to this by becoming angry with his wife who then stopped playing with Rakeem. Rakeem's mother would say a word or two to her husband who by now showed more intense anger and disgust with both his wife and Rakeem. Rakeem's mother viewed the problem, at least in part, as Rakeem being "like a stubborn mule." Rakeem's father viewed the problem as Rakeem being "stupid."

Improving Rakeem's mother's capability and providing her with additional techniques for stimulating Rakeem's language would clearly be insufficient even though this would have seemed like a logical intervention had family interactions been unknown. Access to the the entire family system offered the clinician insights and opportunities for intervention that could not possibly occur in the individual approach. In this case, intervention began with listening to the parents describe their views of the problem and using the counseling techniques of listening, clarifying, tracking, and summarizing. The parents were allowed to talk about the problem without the clinician offering any solutions. Mother demonstrated the techniques she used for stimulating Rakeem and the interactive pattern described above was spontaneously enacted by the parents. We began by commenting positively upon the work of the mother to the father. In other words, as mother played with Rakeem we commented aloud to the father (so that mother could also hear) about what a good job she was doing and how positively Rakeem responded to her visually (looking at her, smiling, showing affection, etc.) even though he did not say words. A noticing assignment was given to the father to pay attention to the different ways in which Rakeem responded positively to his mother at home. As the father began to attend to these positive features of his wife's ability, we quietly began to offer suggestions to mother to increase her effectiveness. This was done in the context of the clinician joining the mother and Rakeem in play. We typically modeled a technique (eg., beginning a phrase and pausing to give Rakeem the opportunity to say the word, but saying it if Rakeem didn't), briefly pointing out what was being done, and asking Rakeem's mother to try it. This increased the opportunities to reward mother for her work and gave new occasions to comment upon her ability to her husband. We frequently framed the latter in terms of how nicely Rakeem *responded* to his mother since this was a visible behavior that the father could see. This new perspective freed the mother to be even more effective since father was developing a new appreciation for what *she* was able to do. At subsequent weekly sessions we evaluated Rakeem's progress in visual attention/alertness (and discussed the positive features of this), his spontaneity of saying words, and his responses to his mother's use of paraphrasing. We worked toward having Rakeem say words to his father. We did not suggest that Rakeem's father play with Rakeem or that he attempt to stimulate language since that clearly was not his role within the family interactive system. While we observed Rakeem's sister's interaction with Rakeem and watched that develop, we did not consciously use her as a resource to help Rakeem since that, too, did not seem consistent with the family's expectations and assignment of roles to male versus female children.

  The interventions used with Rakeem's family show the importance of attending to both simple actions and to interactions. As Rakeem began talking more, it was not possible to link his new behavior with one particular cause. In addition to the above description, there were subtle interventions. We joined with the father by showing appreciation and respect for his success as a businessman. We demonstrated that we viewed male roles differently than he by having the male clinician play with Rakeem. We positively regarded the family as a joined unit. We respected the roles of family members and the hierarchical structure of the family. We acknowledged and tested causal possibilities such as a hearing loss. We became part of the family system. No one intervention, including reinforcing simple actions, could be said to be responsible for changes in Rakeem's expressive language. Further, changes from week to week far exceeded any change that occurred during any of the weekly family sessions.

Steven fifteen years old and severely dysarthric provides another example of the importance of the combination of attention to simple actions and to interactions. His parents were primarily concerned about his noisy eating and secondarily about his speech production. A communicative pattern involving the eating problem repeated itself at mealtimes with Steven's father reacting to Steven's noisy and messy eating by giving him advice to slow down, put less food on the spoon, close his mouth, swallow more frequently, wipe his mouth, participate in conversation between bites, etc. Steven, in turn, ate faster and, therefore, more noisily and messier in response to this "nagging" (to use Steven's term). This resulted in father "nagging" more and finally for mother to become angry with both Steven and her husband. A younger brother sometimes joined the "fray" by making angry comments to his parents or to Steven. The pattern usually ended with each person eating in silence as quickly as possible and leaving the table immediately upon finishing dinner. The simple actions in this case consisted of particular techniques that Steven could use to improve his ability to chew, swallow, reduce the effects of a suckling reflex, maintain lip closure, etc. Interactions related to the problem included the dominant repetitive pattern described above plus others including the parents showing concern for Steven and his problem, Steven's reliance upon his family for support, respect and affection for one another, and constructive efforts to solve the problem.

Steven's parents suggested that the initial goal be for Steven to accept the responsibility for eating as quietly and neatly as he could. This was of some importance to Steven too since he was enrolled in a new school. Some of Steven's peers were reacting to his eating lunch by avoiding the table at which he was sitting. Thus, Steven shared his parents' desire for him to learn to eat as normally as possible. We believed, however, that the dominant interactive pattern was perpetuating the problem and that each family member had too much invested in that pattern to give up the accompanying behavior without specific interventions from us.

Treatment initially focused upon both the dominant repetitive interactive pattern and upon specific techniques for Steven to use when eating. Everyone agreed that the sessions should consist of one clinician working on eating techniques with Steven while the other met with the parents in another room. This symbolized Steven's acceptance of responsibility for helping himself, an appropriate developmental task for a fifteen-year-old, and disengaged the parents from that responsibility. Steven was given written assignments to carry out at mealtimes based upon mobilization points that he described (i.e., things that he knew to do that helped him eat quietly and neatly). Steven brought different types of foods to the first three or four sessions to demonstrate his eating techniques for the clinician to expand upon or modify. Assignments to Steven were based upon these techniques. His parents were not told what Steven was doing. Their assignment during this time began with making neither positive nor negative comments during mealtimes, but to notice anything that they liked and to discuss it with the clinician at the next session. At first, it was difficult for the parents to think of anything that they liked about Steven's eating during the week. As their mealtime experiences were tracked in more depth, they were able to name progressively more positive behaviors. At a brief combined meeting at the third session, Steven's father suggested that it might be good to have table rules which *everyone* in the family was expected to follow. The assignment to the parents was for them to develop and write down rules or guidelines to be discussed at the next session. The rules that they brought to the next week's meeting were discussed jointly by all of us. They were very practical (eg., look at others during mealtime, participate in family conversations, stay at the table until everyone finishes eating, close your mouth when chewing, use your napkin to wipe your mouth, and clear your own dishes from the table) and everyone agreed to attempt to abide by these rules. At this same meeting, during the parents' session, Steven's father suggested that it might be helpful to explain to Steven the nature of his problem and to give the problem a name. We discussed this briefly as a group and agreed that we would all talk about it at the next session, which we did. We named the speech problem as "dysarthria" and described some of the physical characteristics that made it difficult for Steven to eat. These included a suckling reflex, inability to lateralize the tongue and move a bolus of food from side to side, a weak chewing reflex, and hypertonicity and weakness of the lips with protruding upper teeth making it difficult to approximate the lips and to maintain lip closure. We added that it was very difficult for Steven to bite, chew, and move the food in his mouth in preparation for swallowing. Steven especially appreciated hearing this, and his parents, perhaps for the first time, realized the significance of Steven's problem and seemed able to separate lack of motivation from physical difficulty.

After the discussion the family seemed to change in a positive way and we interpreted this as a system transformation or "second order change" (Watzlawick, et al., 1974). A second order change is one in which the structure and basic assumptions of a family system change. This is as opposed to "first order change" which entails only a change in behavior without change in the basic assumptions or structure of the system. At the next session Steven expressed a desire to begin working on speech. His parents said that they didn't feel that they needed to talk about Steven's eating anymore or that it was necessary for them to attend separate sessions each week. Rather, they suggested that they would bring Steven, if he wanted, to work on his speech with his clinician and that once per month we could all meet for a family session. These significant shifts in goals and expectations were symbolic of Steven's growing maturity and were part of the normal adolescent process of becoming increasingly independent. Even though most sessions were to be individual in nature, we began at a different point than we would have had we not involved the family from the beginning.

These two families illustrate a systemic approach to treatment and show how the traditional attention to simple actions may be combined with attention to interactions to facilitate change. The latter could not have been accomplished if the entire family system had not been the unit of treatment.

Improvement occurred in each case, but it was difficult, if not impossible, to attribute the improvement to specific interventions since both simple actions and interactive events were modified. Traditional techniques used by speech-language pathologists were used to change specific speech and eating behaviors (simple actions). Systemic counseling techniques were used to address interactions in which the problematic eating and speech behaviors were embedded.

ASSESSING TREATMENT

We begin with the assumption that we will meet with a family once per week for one hour. Typically, after several sessions the time between sessions is lengthened. Occasionally, individual sessions are added later to supplement the family meetings. The commitment is not to the approach but to changed behavior, and we will do whatever seems necessary in order to evoke or provoke a positive change in communicative behavior.

The typical pattern of a session is as follows: (1) briefly review the goals of treatment; (2) discuss the assignment from the previous week; (3) have family members demonstrate or enact the assignment if it involves use of a behavioral technique; (4) when appropriate, enact the assignment ourselves and experiment with modifying it in order to determine whether this is feasible and would promote further change; (5) have family members carry out the new technique or style of interaction; and, (6) discuss a new assignment. Naturally, not all sessions follow this basic framework. It is, however, a format from which to depart. In this context, the effectiveness of treatment is assessed and modifications are made in the interest of promoting change as quickly as possible.

Review the Goals of Treatment

Family members have already participated in setting treatment goals and have agreed upon them. Their understanding of these, however, is likely to be less complete than that of the clinician since most families are not accustomed to thinking specifically about communicative behavior. Further, the link between the assignment and the goals may not be as clear to families as to the clinician. When the latter seems the case, it is helpful to talk about the goal and the procedures together. For example in a second session we restated the goal as follows, "Our goal is to improve Robert's intelligibility. We all noticed that when he uses more effort, talks louder, and emphasizes the stress and rhythm of his speech that he is much easier to understand. In an effort to encourage him to do this you have been overemphasizing some of the things that you say to him and doing this as you repeat some of the words and phrases that he says to you." In this case, the actual assignment was for the family to notice whether or not these techniques resulted in Robert using more effort, talking louder, and emphasizing the stress and rhythm of his speech. A second assignment was for the family to reinforce Robert when they heard him doing these things.

The example of Robert was taken from the second session with him and his family. Robert had a genetic defect which resulted in mental retardation. He was nine years old. His family included his father; his stepmother; and his stepbrother, the thirteen year old son of his stepmother. Robert lived with this part of his family most of the time. His family also included his natural mother and his mother's friend. Robert visited this part of his family on week-ends. Everyone attended the treatment sessions. All these people were interested in Robert and were willing to help him. Their cooperation and participation was positively framed at the first session in terms of how fortunate Robert was to have so many people who cared about him.

Review the Assignment

It is important to use neutral questioning to learn how family members carry out assignments. At Robert's third session, for example, we asked, "What happened when you exaggerated the rhythm of your speech as you interacted with Robert?" Our assumption was that the assignment had been carried out. Had it not been, family members could have said that they did not do it, that it was unsuccessful, that they modified it, etc. more readily than if our question had been the more accusatory, "Did you do the assignment?" Since it is critical to know the truth about assignments any techniques that lead to elaboration and discussion are useful. The role of the clinician is to match his/her expertise with each family's resources and capabilities in order to effect change in the family member having the communicative problem. This has not been accomplished when the family has not carried out the assignment in any fashion whatsoever. When this occurs it is important to know the reason so that a more appropriate assignment can be given. However, one should not view it as a failure when families change or modify the assignment. The clinician should listen, track, and clarify in order to learn exactly what happened when the assignment was attempted. Once the family's efforts have been explored, they can show the clinician what they did. This gives an even better understanding of the effectiveness of the assignment and allows the clinician to modify it or expand upon it appropriately.

To continue with the example of Robert, his stepmother answered first when we asked what happened when they carried out the assignment. She described many examples of times when she exaggerated the rhythm of her speech. These included when: making cookies with Robert, imitating a person they saw on television, talking with Robert as he arrived home from school each day, putting Robert to bed, eating meals, and interacting in the course of daily living. Tracking was used to learn exactly what happened in terms of their location in the house, what each person said in the dialog, how each reacted emotionally to the assignment in terms of ease and enjoyment, and the extent to which Robert changed his speech during the interaction. Other examples were given by Robert's father and his step-brother. Robert's natural mother modified the assignment slightly in order to make it fit her activities with her son. She carried out the assignment when singing songs with Robert and when reading books to him. She described exactly what had happened and we asked her to look at a book with Robert during the session and show us what she did. While requests for enactments could be interpreted as skepticism on the clinician's part, when this is done out of genuine curiosity and interest we have not found families to be defensive. More often, they enjoy showing us what they have done. Those interactions that look especially favorable are rewarded. When young children are involved, we particularly like to reward a parent by reacting positively to the parent-child relationship in terms of the child's response to the parent and/or the parent's particular manner of interacting with the child. We also reward family behavior that shows enjoyment of communicating and interacting with the client. This is done by talking about the positive things we notice.

Enact the Assignment and Develop a New One

After Robert's family members described their activities and enacted the assignment, we interacted with Robert and began experimenting by calling Robert's attention to specific sounds and sound groups while emphasizing the rhythm of speech. Since Robert did not always close his lips for bilabial sounds and because exaggerating the rhythm of speech seemed to facilitate lip closure, several minutes were spent in an effort to determine the feasibility of an assignment that would incorporate attending particularly to bilabial sounds in the context of increased loudness and rhythm. We practiced words such as "mama, mine, boy, pie." Robert's family began adding words that they knew would come up during the week and we discussed the possibility of adding a list of specific words containing /b/, /p/, and /m/ to the assignment of overall exaggerated use of loudness variation and rhythm. Robert's family began asking Robert to imitate family-related words (i.e., words associated with family experiences). This gave us the opportunity to observe how such an assignment would be carried out at home. His family members rewarded Robert's attempts appropriately and we commented about the importance of doing this and their ability to do so. We discussed whether or not attending to all three phonemes would be too difficult for Robert and for the family and decided that it would not be. A list of ten words and phrases based upon words said at home was developed for practice. Correct imitation was defined as lip approximation and was to be rewarded. The previous week's assignment was also continued since it had been successful in improving Robert's intelligibility.

It was suggested that the ten specific words be practiced during normal everyday activities. A "stop and say" activity which we have used successfully with a number of families was described. In this activity, the practice word is said to the client by a family member in the course of natural interactions such as when eating dinner, when entering the same room, while watching television, etc. The family member says the word, the family member with the speech-language problem repeats it, success is rewarded, and natural activities are resumed. Most families make an enjoyable activity out of this and find it to be an easy way to incorporate structured speech into everyday events. In addition, since the word list contained words and phrases that were known to be part of family conversation, it was expected that use of the words would arise out of natural interactions.

CONCLUSION

The activities described above provide an example of the manner in which treatment effectiveness can be assessed each week. When an assignment has not been carried out, neutral questioning should be used to determine what happened. The family should then be invited to participate in developing a more appropriate assignment. The new assignment should be one that family members can do, one that fits the lifestyle of the family, and one that will be effective in changing speech-language behavior. In addition, periodic language samples, re-testing, review of previously made audio and video tapes from home or the clinic, and use of assignments assessing progress are used to determine the effectiveness of treatment. In our experience, when family members participate in assessing the results of what they are doing there is less likelihood that ineffective procedures will be continued beyond a week or two. Family members usually know whether or not their activities are promoting change and are eager to alter them when they are not. When families are allowed to be full participants on the treatment team both the clinician and family members are freed to communicate honestly and respectfully about the value of treatment procedures.

CHAPTER 8

TERMINATION AND LINKAGE

A decision to end family treatment must be made at some point in the Family Based Treatment process. We have used four different options as we have ended therapy with our families: a last session scheduled at the end of a predetermined number of sessions; a gradual spacing of sessions leading to a mutual decision to terminate as family members assume responsibility for intervention; termination following a one or two session consultation; and linking to other professionals who continue treatment with the client. A combination of methods is sometimes used since other professionals may be involved following termination of family meetings.

Defined Number of Sessions

For various reasons, the clinician and family may agree on a defined number of sessions with a termination point determined at the outset. Summer sessions with children who will be returning to school services in the fall, treatment at short and long-term medical facilities that ends when the patient is transferred to another facility or goes home, and a limited number of family sessions organized to fit the busy schedules of the participants are examples of situations that require a predetermined ending. This kind of termination may be as dependent on the clinician's professional options as it is on the family's availability. At the final session, accomplishments are highlighted and the family members are complimented for their participation. When the client will be continuing services with another speech-language pathologist, we include that person in the final session so that a smooth transition is assured.

Gradual Spacing of Sessions

When families are empowered participants in treatment, it is not unusual to reduce the frequency of meetings after several sessions and after the clinician is confident that family members are intervening effectively. This is especially true when the communicative disorder is one that is expected to change through a combination of treatment and maturation and change occurs slowly. Complete termination of treatment is usually inappropriate in such cases and may be replaced with bi-weekly or monthly sessions with the family. Even longer intervals may be planned as treatment progresses and the clinician assures mutual accessibility with the family. An important aspect of such a decision is that it be made mutually with the family. We often call the longer break a "vacation" and schedule a follow-up meeting four to six months after the last regular meeting so that progress can be monitored.

It is significant to note that treatment interventions are continuing during this time even though the speech-language pathologist is not meeting with the family. The family has learned to build speech-language change into its everyday life and is maintaining the gains achieved during family treatment. The "signal" that such a change in scheduling might be appropriate is that the clinician finds that the creative strategizing process does not lead to a significant alteration in the assignments. Naturally, the clinician assumes that family members are continuing to intervene during these breaks. This is a valid assumption in nearly every case since family members are an integral part of the solution-focused treatment team. A follow-up meeting monitors progress and can also be used to evaluate developmental change and the possibility of another series of sessions.

One or Two Session Consultation

Many clinicians have heavy caseloads and are not able to work with families on an ongoing basis. One or two consultation sessions are then arranged with families so that the clinician's schedule does not become overcrowded. A school conference is an example of this kind of meeting. Even though the time is short, the Family Based Treatment process and techniques may be used and the families are enlisted to join the habilitative team.

In addition, clinicians who work systemically are likely to be called upon by families for one or two-session consultations. Families who request this are not seeking assessment and treatment in the usual sense; rather, they want the speech-language pathologist's opinion about a communicative problem and/or suggestions for ways to improve interaction with a family member having a communicative disorder. Termination of services is expected after the number of agreed-upon sessions has been completed.

Linking With Other Professionals

The process of linking with other professionals is as much a method of treatment as are the usual interventions related to behavior change. It is not unusual for several professionals and even several speech-language pathologists to become involved when treatment begins with a very young child. Over time, the treatment team may expand to include many different teachers, school and clinical psychologists, parent interventionists, occupational therapists, physical therapists, school administrators, rehabilitation counselors, social workers, and speech-language pathologists.

Treatment becomes significantly more complicated as the need to share and integrate data expands with the addition of each new professional. The speech-language pathologist's treatment in many of these cases should include linking the families with other professionals in a way that advances and maintains the families as integral decision-makers on the treatment team. The speech-language pathologist can facilitate this process in several ways. These include showing that he/she hears and respects the family's views, talking about the communicative problem as it manifests itself interactively, describing the interventions that family members have carried out, and having family members demonstrate their skills to team members.

The clinician must also respect the views of the other professionals on the team. A systemic approach accommodates different views and is necessary to the successful functioning of treatment teams.

SUMMARY

Four different options have been described relative to ending Family Based Treatment. Two of these are variations of agreed-upon or implied short-term treatment or consultation. Not all families with a member with a communicative disorder need or desire more than a few sessions with a speech-language pathologist. In some cases a family may want the opinion of the speech-language pathologist about the severity of a problem, the need for treatment, or about suggestions for activities that could be carried out at home. With other families, services are more traditionally oriented and termination is not pre-determined. When treatment is long-term and the client is young, maturation may be a factor in change and breaks in treatment may be arranged. When services are to be provided by another professional person, it is important to link the family with the appropriate person or persons and clarify the anticipated level of family participation.

CHAPTER 9

COUNSELING TECHNIQUES

Family participation in the treatment of communicative disorders is most effective when counseling techniques are integrated into the entire treatment process. One should not think of counseling as an adjunct to therapy set aside as a separate process from the evaluation and treatment of speech-language-hearing problems. Rather, we suggest that counseling be defined as the use of a set of techniques that enables the clinician to respond to client and family statements, behaviors, and interactions in a manner that expands clinical effectiveness and, therefore, also enhances change. In this chapter we will describe the specific techniques that are used in working with families, discuss the integrated use of counseling techniques, and outline the issues associated with the grief process that are relevant to Family Based Treatment.

USING THE TECHNIQUES

The techniques described here are used by family therapists, speech-language pathologists, children, parents, spouses, counselors, psychologists, teachers, business people,

---

Material in this chapter is adapted with permission from Andrews, M.A., Application of Family Therapy Techniques to the Treatment of Language Disorders, in *Seminars in Speech and Language,* Volume 7, Number 4, New York, 1986, Thieme Medical Publishers, Inc.

grandparents and all manner of human beings who want to interact successfully with clients, family members and co-workers. These techniques have usually been identified, described and taught by counseling professionals but are not owned by them and may be used by any person who finds pleasure in initiating creative change-producing human contact. We will describe these techniques as we have used them and encourage the reader to be adventurous and creative in adapting them to his/her own personal style.

Joining

The speech-language pathologist gains acceptance of and admittance into the family system through the process of joining. This is accomplished by acknowledging and promoting the family's strengths, respecting the established roles of family members, and by affirming the self-worth of each individual (Simon, et al., 1985). As the joining process evolves, family members begin to know that the clinician understands and respects each person's point of view. This accommodation to the family's perspective promotes a willingness on the part of family members to hear and understand the clinician's professional ideas regarding treatment. Joining becomes a reciprocally beneficial process that creates a context for cooperation.

The joining process begins with the first telephone or in-person contact and continues into the first and subsequent family meetings. Most professionals experience a sense of excitement, some trepidation, and genuine interest in wanting to get to know this new family group. As the first meeting begins, the clinician listens respectfully, responds nonjudgmentally, and begins to experience the concerns, struggles, satisfactions, and hopes that the family members bring to the session. The clinician also begins to understand what the family members are saying about their view of reality (Minuchin, 1974). An early sign that the joining process is underway occurs when the family agrees to work with the clinician in future sessions. As treatment continues, the family and clinician interact in an increasingly cooperative manner. A trusting alliance is formed that facilitates joint decision-making and positive change in the family environment of the person with a communicative disorder. Gradually, a bond is established that assures the family's continued participation in the habilitation process.

Behaviors that may be adopted to facilitate the joining process are socializing about everyday issues, mirroring the posture of the person being listened to, using language and terminology that matches the family's level of understanding, matching affect (smiling, frowning, looking puzzled), and identifying each family member's unique interests and attributes. Most of these behaviors evolve quite naturally when the professional is committed to an appreciation of the family members' and client's points of view.

Attending

Attending is conveyed through posturing and is a part of the listening and clarifying process (Rogers, 1965). In order to attend fully to each member of the family, the clinician positions him/herself so that eye contact is possible with each family member. Chairs should be arranged, for example, in a circle with toys, manuals, and other equipment placed on a side table next to the clinician. Attention to each person's verbal and nonverbal communication is shown through cues such as eye contact, nodding of the head, naturally friendly facial expressions, and an open-body position. A strong desire to understand each person's thoughts, feelings, hopes, and fears regarding the communicative problem should be experienced by the clinician. This desire tends to be conveyed to the family and, in turn, helps to relax family members. The family invariably responds positively to an attentive, concerned professional.

Clarification

The content and communicative intent of the speaker's verbal and nonverbal expressions become clear as the clinician attends to each family member, accepts silence to allow the speaker an opportunity to think about responses, nods and utters an occasional "mm-hm," and restates what the speaker has said. Each of these responses conveys to the speaker, "I am listening to you very carefully" (Benjamin, 1981).

Clarification is the interviewer's restatement for the interviewee of what the latter has said or tried to say (Benjamin, 1981). The response may be simplified to make it clearer and more understandable but the meaning and intent expressed by the speaker should always be maintained. The goal is to develop a clear understanding of the speaker's perspective while also helping the speaker to clarify his/her own ideas. Clarification encourages the speaker to continue and also promotes the joining process. The following is an example of clarification as it was used with a family having a language-delayed child.

Father: Whenever I try to get him to talk to me he just doesn't say anything. . . . ummm. . . Carol (his wife, who is also present) can at least get him to make some kind of, uh, sound or use motions with his hands.

Clinician: You've really tried hard to get him to talk. . but. . .just haven't had much luck with that. Carol seems to be able to get him to respond a little more easily.

Father: Yeh, I don't know if he doesn't hear me or. . . . if he's just stubborn, or maybe I'm talking to him wrong, or something. . . . .

Clinician: It sounds like you've thought of lots of things that might be making this a problem and it seems like you'd really like to figure out what's going on here.

> Father: Yeh, we came here today because we thought you could help with that. What do you think is wrong?
>
> Clinician: (responding directly to the father's question, discontinuing clarification) O.K., that's a good question. As we work together and learn about what you and Carol have noticed. . . and as I do a speech-language assessment. . . I think we should be able to find some answers to this problem.

Useful information was gleaned from this brief bit of clarification. The clinician learned that the father is concerned, has tried unsuccessfully to elicit speech and language, and is seeking help from an "expert." The clinician indicated that she understood his perspective, used language of participation, joined him in his quest for "answers," and reiterated that the parents and clinician would operate as a team as the language delay is assessed and treated. At this early stage, care was taken to resist becoming the "answer person." Instead, the clinician indicated that further exploration of the problem was necessary.

Clarification is a useful interviewing skill because family members will let the clinician know if he/she has missed the intent of what is being said, thus offering opportunity to restate in a different way. For example, imagine resuming the clarification sequence during the second interchange. Notice that the interchange takes a different twist as the father corrects a clarification statement that was not quite on target.

> Clinician: You've thought of lots of things that might be making this a problem and it seems like you'd really like to figure out what's going on here.
>
> Father: Well no, I. . uh. . . really don't have any idea about what the problem could be. I don't care what's causing this thing with Chris I just want to *do* something about it.

Clinician: O.K., the causes aren't important to you but you're eager to get something started.

Father: Yeh, he's already three years old and should be talking by now. I just want to know what we can do!

Clinician: (responding directly to the father's statement, discontinuing clarification) Good, I want to get Carol's ideas now, then do a speech-language assessment, and then we'll figure out something that we all can do to help us solve this problem.

A different initial understanding has been gathered from the changed interaction between the father and the clinician. The first exchange indicated a desire for "answers" and the second a desire for "action." This understanding of the father's perspective will help the clinician strategize for change and design an appropriate assignment. Another important benefit that has been derived from either exchange is that the father has begun to sense that he is dealing with a professional that respects his opinions and is willing to accommodate his concerns for his son.

Reflection

Reflection, a skill described by Carl Rogers (Rogers, 1965), is similar to clarification but also includes the restatement of feelings in order to help the individual access the deeper meanings being expressed. Roger's model proposes that when this technique is used, along with unconditional positive regard, individuals are able to sort out and solve vexing problems using their own personal resources. Many of the problems that families must face when their member has a communicative disorder do not have clear-cut solutions. Furthermore, when professionals tell family members how they *should* feel (e.g. "don"t feel bad, everything will be O.K." or, "you shouldn't be saying things like that, it will make

Sarah feel worse") feelings are denied and potential personal resources are buried within the individual. Instead, when the speech-language pathologist responds to expressions of feelings, the joining process is enhanced and family members are given permission to deal with the frustration, pain, and confusion that they are experiencing, thus eventually uncovering their own solutions to idiosyncratic problems.

The clinician can use reflection when strong feelings are being expressed and/or when the feeling content of the speaker's statements is evident. This is likely to happen when the family is experiencing a crisis associated with a communicative handicap such as might occur with diagnosis of hearing loss, a serious head trauma, the birth of a child with a cleft lip, or a stroke resulting in aphasia. Strong feelings also may be expressed as family members show anger, disappointment, sorrow, happiness, confusion, exhaustion, etc. related to difficulties that may seem less serious to the professional. When the communicative disorder is associated with a permanent disability these feelings, particularly anger, may appear to be directed at the clinician. Understanding that the feelings are directed at the unfairness of the disability itself and at the family's perplexing and painful situation will help the professional respond appropriately with reflective listening.

Reflection may also be used in noncrisis situations once a relationship has been established between the client and family members. Some clinicians, however, are comfortable with expressions of feelings and use reflection during the first family meeting even if it is not a crisis situation. The success of this technique, early in treatment, depends upon the clinician's intent. If the intent is to show respect and understanding and to clearly reflect what is being said, even when this is different from what the clinician thinks should be said or felt, the technique is likely to enhance clinician-family cooperation. The clinician's decision to use reflection will depend upon the strength of the emotions being expressed and personal comfort with the technique. As with clarification, the speaker will correct the clinician if the reflection is off-target but will continue to express him/herself knowing that an effort is being made to understand the feelings and ideas being shared. Our experience has been that a few reflective statements help release the emotional pain being expressed. Family members let us know when they are ready to continue efforts directed toward speech-language change, knowing that the clinician understands their need to deal with these feelings while work continues.

The following excerpt continues the interview begun earlier and shows the use of reflective listening during a first session:

> Clinician: Carol, John's noticed that you can get Chris to talk to you and to use motions from time to time. Can you tell me more about this?
>
> Mother: Well. . . . . . I suppose he does use more sounds when he's with me, but I get so tired of trying to get him to say something and sometimes just get mad because I think he *could* do a lot more than he tries to do and I don't like it when he uses motions because I think that's just an excuse not to talk.
>
> Clinician: It sounds like you get pretty upset and. . maybe . . just feel like giving up sometimes because Chris doesn't want to try to talk to you.
>
> Mother: Yeh. . . . . . He's really not a bad kid but it's so hard to know what he wants when he starts to holler, or turns away from me, or gives up trying. I. . . . I . . . don't think he means to be so stubborn because sometimes he starts to cry when I get upset with him and then he hangs on me like he's afraid I'm going to leave him or something like that. I'm almost at my wits end with all of this.
>
> Clinician: Mm. . .hm. . .this problem is bothering you a lot and you'd really like to figure out how to get Chris to try to respond to you so you two could maybe enjoy each other a little bit. . . . . instead of always feeling so frustrated.

Mother: Oh, yeh. . . . . that would sure be nice but I don't have a clue about how to get it to happen.

Clinician: O.K. . . . . .this whole thing has been tough for you and John (husband) and you both want to figure out what can be done to motivate Chris to talk more. I'd like to ask a few more questions about what you two have noticed and then we'll move on to figuring out what we can *do*. Does that seem O.K. with you?

Mother: Sure, I'll try *anything* to get him talking.

The use of reflection helped mother express her frustration and also let her know that the clinician was comfortable with the feeling statements that are a natural part of a family's response to a communicative disorder. Incidentally, more data were gathered about mother's interactive responses to Chris' language delay. Since many of their interchanges ended in conflict, and this was frustrating to both of them, it was learned that mother would like to experience a decrease in this kind of interaction. Again, reflection was discontinued when mother seemed, in this communicative interchange, to be finished expressing feelings. The clinician, however, continued to indicate that solving the problem required a joint effort and that the family's thoughts and ideas were respected and important.

Not all family members express feelings and not all clinicians are able to respond reflectively to family members who do express deeper emotions. Nevertheless, reflection is a useful skill to cultivate since its occasional use will open the interactive treatment process to greater understanding, empathy, and change. Reflection, clarification, and creative strategizing are not mutually exclusive activities. These interconnected skills are used to move the treatment process in the direction of cooperative efforts aimed at establishing clear goals and procedures relative to speech-language change.

Summarizing

Summary statements are made at transition points and at the end of each session. For example, when the family interview portion of the first session is completed, the clinician should summarize what has been said. "You, Dad, want to *do* something about Chris' talking problem. Mom, you're sometimes at your wits end and get pretty discouraged but still have enough energy to try something else. You're both really anxious to get some change in Chris' communication and hope that I will be able to offer ideas that will help. Does this about sum up what you have told me so far?"

The clinician should always remember to use language that matches the family's language level and the summary must continue to show sensitivity to that issue. Verbal summaries assure that the family members and clinician understand the various points of view that are being expressed. The anticipation and act of summarizing helps the clinician organize and remember important data related to the family's perspective of the speech-language problem.

Tracking Interactive Patterns

Tracking is a technique described by Minuchin (1974) who uses it as part of the joining process to help the family and clinician develop an understanding of the family's structure. Our use of tracking is focused on identifying family resources rather than family structure. We track a family's interactive patterns in two ways. First, by asking neutral questions and then using clarifying statements in response to these questions, we learn about family responses to communicative events as these occur in sequences of behavior. As we attend to the family members' descriptions of interactive events, communicative sequences are identified and new information about the contextual issues surrounding the problem are discovered. Second, we observe family interaction as it spontaneously occurs in the session, or we request an enactment (Minuchin, 1974) in order to observe spontaneous interaction relating to the communicative disorder.

Questions are asked from a position of neutrality (Fleuridas, et al., 1986; Tomm, 1988). This means that the clinician is nonjudgmental in the approach to each person and does not "side" with any one family member. Questions must not be disguised statements but are exploratory in nature and are asked with an attitude of respect, curiosity, and an intense desire to learn how the family interacts around issues associated with the communicative disorder. Questions asked in this way elicit important data that are then used when creatively strategizing for change.

In addition, the new thinking that is generated by such questioning creates a systemic perspective. This perspective interfaces with an appreciation for the interconnectedness of family interaction related to the communicative disorder. Family members and clinicians alike gain new insights as questioning proceeds. The family member's response to each question influences the clinician's clarification of the response and the formation of the next question. Each interview is a unique, idiosyncratic event created and shaped by the clinician's responses to family members and provides a rich array of data to be used in strategizing for change. The following excerpt shows how questions asked from a neutral position facilitate the tracking process:

> Clinician: Carol, you said that there are many times when you try to help Chris talk. Can you tell me what happened the last time you did that?
>
> Mother: Well . . . . it's hard to remember an exact time.
>
> Father: . . . . what about when you're in the kitchen trying to get something cooked and he's in there fussing and carrying on and you can't figure out what he's saying?
>
> Mother: Yeh . . . . that seems to happen every day . . . and . . . yeh, that happened last night. I was really in a

hurry because I'd just gotten home from work and John, you were trying to pick up the house and Chris was fussy . . . . . seems like he's usually fussy at night . . and he was trying to tell me something, I think, but I couldn't figure it out at all.

Clinician: O.K. . . this is a good everyday example . . . that's what we want to look at. So . . . you're in the kitchen trying to fix something to eat, John's picking up the house . . . .

Mother: . . . . . Yeh . . . . and don't forget Samantha's (10 month old daughter) also fussing because she's hungry too.

Clinician: O.K. . . things are pretty hectic for everyone right then and in the midst of all this Chris is wanting to communicate something and you can't figure it out at all. What do you do?

Mother: Well, I usually stop what I'm doing and look at him and say, "Tell me again, I can't understand you!"

Clinician: What happens then?

Mother: He makes those sounds again and I keep trying to figure it out.

Clinician: How do you try to figure it out? What do you do?

Mother: Well . . . . sometimes I can tell what he's trying to say because he's pointing at something, usually some kind of food, so I might say, "cracker, is that what you want, a cracker?"

Clinician: When you ask him if he wants a cracker, as he's pointing in the direction of the crackers, how does he respond?

Mother: Well . . . . if I've guessed right, he nods his head and then I usually give him a cracker and he's happy for a few minutes. If I guessed wrong, he hollers louder and I keep on trying to figure out what he's trying to say. After two or three guesses, I give up and he starts crying and runs to John and John starts to play with him or something like that.

Clinician: So when Chris is trying to tell you something and you can figure it out from his motions and sounds, he's happy for a little while. If you can't figure it out, he keeps trying and sometimes cries and if John's around runs to him.

Mother: Uh huh . . . . that's about it.

Clinician: John, is this about how you see it happening too?

Father: Yep, except I don't even try to figure out what he's saying because it's impossible for me.

Clinician: What do you do instead?

Father: Usually, I'll try to play with him or something so he'll quiet down so Carol can finish cooking because I'm pretty hungry by then! (John and Carol both laugh at John's joke, look at each other and smile as they seem to be sharing their mutual frustration).

This brief tracking excerpt elicited a great deal of helpful information. Chris appears to have a clear desire to communicate with his mother but is unable to do so in a manner that is rewarding to the two of them. Mother has the ability to figure out Chris' meaning even when under considerable stress and father is willing to help out when things become hectic relative to Chris' behavior. In addition, the nonverbal alliance shown by Chris' parents indicated that they support one another during the stressful times associated with normal daily living. Although additional tracking and the speech-language assessment are yet to occur, the clinician can begin to formulate a hypothesis about this particular family's resources and can fit those resources to an appropriate first step relative to speech-language change.

Tracking is *not* done to figure out what is wrong with the family. It is done to uncover interactive patterns, particularly those that can be accessed for change and then used to treat the communicative disorder. This example shows a determined and resourceful child, a creative mother who can "figure things out," and a father willing to be supportive and wanting to "do something." Mother and father seem to enjoy a friendly relationship despite their difficulties and show an ability to cooperate with one another and with the clinician. These resources will be very useful as the clinician and family continue their quest for change.

A second kind of tracking occurs when family members enact spontaneous examples of interactive events. For example, when an adult daughter begins to communicate with her aphasic mother, a brother plays with his language-delayed sister, or a father discusses a problem with his head-injured teenager, the clinician will want to observe this behavior to see how family members interact with the person with the communicative disorder. If spontaneous events do not occur, the clinician can ask family members to discuss an issue, read a book to a child, play a game with an adolescent, etc. making certain that the activity is within the framework of the family's ability and understanding. We often request enactments in follow-up sessions as a way of observing the family's integration of new behaviors into their natural style. Usually, during early sessions, the family is more comfortable showing spontaneous interactions. The clinician's job is to allow these to take place without interfering.

Tracking helps the clinician gather data about the interactive patterns in which the communicative disorder is embedded. These data are "stored" in the clinicians mental file of information and will be used to appropriately link the family's idiosyncratic style to desired speech-language changes. As this process evolves, attention is paid to the useful resources that are uncovered since these must be reinforced and appreciated. The clinician may also notice behaviors that may be reinforcing the persistence of the problem, but those will be intentionally ignored as positive behaviors are discovered, strengthened, and reinforced. The tracking process also helps family members, themselves, uncover attributes and ideas that lead to changed behaviors. As they think about the interactive events related to their family member's communicative disorder in new and different ways, they tend to acquire insights heretofore unexplored.

Creative Strategizing

As the family session continues, the clinician and family develop an understanding of the problem as it is experienced in the natural context. They are joined in their desire for positive change; patterns of interaction in which the problem is embedded have been identified; and clinical testing has occurred (see chapter 4). The clinician-client-family team must now use this information to create change.

Creative strategizing, the process that initiates this change, has been adapted from the work of strategic family therapists (Haley, 1976; Madanes, 1981). "Strategic therapists set clear goals which always include solving the presenting problem. The emphasis is not on a method to be applied to all cases but on designing a strategy for each specific problem. Since the therapy focuses on the social context of human dilemmas, the therapist's task is to design an intervention in the client's social situation" (Madanes, 1981, p.19). Creative strategizing, as we use it, begins as the clinician starts to formulate hypotheses about the family's interactive resources and connects these strengths to desired speech-language change. Creative strategizing culminates in a simple, yet effective assignment that is discussed and, if necessary, refined with the family's input.

The speech-language pathologist begins the creative

strategizing process at the time of the first family contact and continues to think about strategies for change as information is gathered and summarized. Strategizing focuses on creating task assignments that will facilitate speech-language change. Care is taken to design assignments that encourage family members to maintain their established roles while respecting their view of reality. Creative strategizing "flavors" the entire treatment process and is the result of the joining of the clinician's expertise with the family's idiosyncratic style in a continuously evolving manner. This nudges the therapeutic system in the direction of positive speech-language change. This change is concretely identified in the goals and procedures that are outlined and discussed at each session.

Task Assignment

According to Haley (1976), there are three purposes to assigning tasks. These are to encourage people to behave differently, to intensify the relationship with the therapist, and to gather information. With this in mind, the outcome of a task assignment is never considered a failure. Careful tracking of behavior surrounding attempts to implement an assignment provides the clinician and family with new data regarding the communicative disorder and informs the creative strategizing process so that new assignments may be developed. Two skills aid us in assigning tasks: the use of a compliment and an egalitarian assignment delivery.

First, we find that the use of a compliment is an excellent prelude to the delivery of the task. deShazer (1985) and his team of family therapists describe the therapeutic use of the compliment and make it a powerful part of their model for family and individual change. The speech-language pathologist's compliment to each family may be directed to the family as a whole or to individual family members but should always be based on information gathered during the family interview portion of the session. Compliments may be general such as, "We are very impressed by your willingness to find a time when all of you could meet to help us figure out how best to help your mother. Your concern for her is clearly evident" (delivered to the adult children and their spouses of a 78 year old woman with global aphasia). Or, the compliment can be specific to family members. For example, "Sean (8 year old brother of language delayed 4 year old female), we noticed that you played with Jennifer very nicely tonight. You listened to everything she said and even repeated some of the words she used to show her that you understood her. That was very good! . . . . . Mom, your expansion of Jennifer's sentences is impressive. When Jennifer says, 'cookie gone', you respond with, 'The cookie's gone, the cookie's all gone.' That's excellent. We think her progress is related to your remembering to do this . . . . Dad, you continue to play with Jennifer in an attentive, calm way . . . . . this helps her attend to the activity at hand as well as to your talking together. Keep up the good work. Now, let's think about adding something new to our efforts. This week we'd like you to try_____" The clinician can also write a brief compliment on the family's assignment sheet.

With the eventual delivery of a compliment in mind, the professional "tunes in" to the family's resources and this effort becomes part of the creative strategizing process. The compliment also paves the way for the family's acceptance of the assignment which, of course, is designed to fit their ability to cooperate in the treatment process. The compliment also helps the family become more comfortable with their role on the treatment team. Unfortunately, many families seem to expect criticism and informal lectures about what they are doing wrong. When this does not happen, and an honest compliment is delivered instead, they become empowered to participate in a more cooperative and active manner. The compliment is derived from the clinician's honest appraisal of the family's resources and should never be phony. With some families, compliments are easy to give and one can readily choose from several options. With other families a concerted effort must be made to find appropriate compliments, but one can always be found.

Second, (as described in chapter 6) the task must be carefully linked to the family's resources and should be delivered in an egalitarian manner. The task assignment may be prefaced with phrases such as, "How about trying _____"; "Since it seemed to help Sarah when I did_____, what do you think of your trying _____?"; I wonder what you think of this idea. . . . . . . ?" This kind of delivery demonstrates equality and continues to emphasize the importance of a cooperative relationship between the clinician and the family. When the assignment is framed in an egalitarian way and is carefully designed to connect family resources to the desired speech-language changes, it is almost always accepted. Modifications and changes suggested by the family are welcomed, and these are used to make the assignment more closely "fit" their ability to cooperate.

AN INTEGRATED APPROACH TO COUNSELING

When counseling techniques are integrated into speech-language treatment, the benefits that are obtained permeate the entire treatment process. A metaphor that describes this perspective is derived from the consideration of preparing a subtly flavored tomato sauce to be served with fresh pasta. When basil is added to the sauce it does not settle in one area and affect only that part of the sauce; instead, it permeates the entire culinary creation and changes the flavor of the sauce as well as the pasta-sauce final product. Counseling techniques are not added to the treatment process at various points and then ignored as work continues. Rather, the clinician's continuing use of these techniques "flavors" the treatment process in a way that changes the totality of the clinician-family relationship and profoundly effects the outcome of treatment. Furthermore, these techniques are not reserved for "problem situations" but are clinical skills that enhance the ongoing work of speech-language pathologists as they use their clinical expertise to create change for their clients and their family members.

The specific events and times that require the use of counseling techniques cannot always be anticipated; however, there are several treatment situations that may lead the clinician to integrate the techniques into the treatment process. These include enlisting family cooperation and participation; interviewing clients and family members to obtain diagnostic and other information; presenting assessment results, especially unwelcome information; responding to emotions that are expressed by clients and/or family members; communicating with co-workers, supervisors, and supervisees; and problem solving with professionals from different treatment orientations. A discussion of each of these situations follows.

Enlisting Family Cooperation and Participation

Most family members approach the clinician and the family treatment experience showing a comfortable ability to cooperate and to join the treatment team. This ability is enhanced as the clinician uses appropriate listening and creative strategizing skills. Some family members, however, may show disinterest, hostility, or other emotions and behaviors that seem to signal an unwillingness to participate. These behaviors change as the clinician joins the family, listens empathically, and shows respect for the divergent views expressed. Many of the families referred to us had been identified as "uncooperative" by one or more professionals. The use of counseling techniques along with the assumption that each family member cared deeply for his/her member with a communicative disorder helped us uncover the family's unique style of cooperating. The idea that every family has an ability to cooperate is described in the work of deShazer (1985). deShazer and his team of family therapists discover the family's style of cooperating by analyzing the responses of their clients to assigned tasks and then creating subsequent tasks that more closely approximate the family's response. The team's assumption is that if family members do not cooperate with the therapist, the therapist has failed to develop a task that fits the family's style of cooperating. The team must then request behavior that is more isomorphic to the family's patterns. Speech-language pathologists who practice joining, clarifying, reflecting, and creative strategizing will be able to enlist family cooperation as they understand and connect with the family's view of reality.

Interviewing Clients and Family Members to Obtain Diagnostic And Other Information

Interviewing techniques are important additions to the clinician's repertoire of counseling skills. Clarifying, reflecting, neutral questioning, and summarizing elicit and organize information in a way that greatly enhances the clinician's ability to link the family's style of cooperating to the speech-language changes that are desired. A well conducted interview generates a reciprocal flow of information and creates a mutual understanding of the problems to be solved. Often, new ideas related to treatment options also emerge as clinician, client, and family members uncover unexpected resources. These interviewing techniques are critical to the successful outcome of a first meeting and are also used as progress is assessed and as therapy continues.

Presenting Assessment Results, Especially Unwelcome Information

Speech-language pathologists and audiologists are sometimes confronted with the unpleasant task of informing clients and family members of assessment results that are difficult to share because the information is unwelcome. Presenting audiometric results that confirm the suspected profound hearing loss of a two-year-old, explaining the results of a receptive language test that place a developmentally delayed four-year-old below the first percentile, sharing the cognitive assessment results with a family following their twenty-year-old son's severe head trauma, and explaining to adult children that their beloved mother's global aphasia may be irreversible, are examples that are not unfamiliar to speech-language pathologists and audiologists. Understanding the importance of presenting information in it's simplest form when the crisis is new, yet continuing to share an honest professional perspective as the therapeutic relationship evolves, requires the use of counseling techniques. As the clinician responds to the client and family members' verbal and nonverbal reactions to undesirable information, the techniques of empathic listening, clarifying, reflecting, and summarizing are used. In addition, the clinician's knowledge of the grief process enables sensitive and appropriate use of these skills.

Responding to Expressions of Emotion

Communicative disorders naturally create an array of feelings that may be expressed by the client and/or family members. These feelings may be different for each family member, and if the disorder is associated with a permanent disability, will emerge, disappear, and re-emerge throughout the family life cycle. Expression of these feelings is a normal part of the adaptation to the problem and should be viewed as natural and acceptable by the clinician. When the clinician or other professionals associated with the client and family attempt to ignore and or disqualify these feelings (e.g., "Don't be upset, we'll get some hearing aids on Johnny, and then we can teach him to talk"), the family's *normal* grief process may be subverted in a way that will be detrimental to treatment. Honest expression of feelings must be acknowledged and supported in order for families to engage in the serious work of treatment. Further, referral to a psychologist or counselor may be unnecessary and even compound the problem in some cases. Family members who had been referred for counseling by other professionals have told us of thinking, "Now, in addition to all I am going through, I have been referred to *another* counselor. There must be something really wrong with me." Most families do not need additional psychological counseling when the clinician is able to accept and respond appropriately to tears, anger, depression, and other *normal* expressions of feeling. The calm presence of an empathic clinician who uses reflection and neutral questioning can be expected to benefit clients and family members as they express the emotions created by the circumstances associated with a communicative disorder.

Communicating With Co-Workers, Supervisors and Supervisees

Speech-language pathologists and audiologists work together in many capacities as students, professors, supervisors, and as equal members on treatment teams. A common interest in learning about and treating communicative disorders unites them in their work. Nevertheless, differences sometimes emerge and problem solving is desirable as these differences are assessed and solutions are developed. When at least one member of the dyad or group in question is able to use counseling techniques, problems can be identified and solved with greater ease than when these skills are not accessed. If more than one person is able to use clarifying, neutral questioning, summarizing, and assigning tasks, excellent solutions tend to emerge quickly and easily.

Communicating With Professionals From Different Treatment Orientations

Many speech-language pathologists and audiologists are members of treatment teams composed of professionals with varying responsibilities relative to communicatively disordered persons and their families. Each member of this professional system is concerned about the well-being of clients and has a different perspective of treatment. The use of counseling techniques will help the speech-language pathologist maintain a polyocular view, assess the resources that are available, and cooperate in developing effective treatment plans. We believe, of course, that the clients' family members should also be equal partners in this treatment planning. Clarifying, summarizing, creative strategizing, and task assignment are particularly useful techniques that can be used during team meetings.

UNDERSTANDING THE GRIEVING AND LOSS PROCESS

When working with families in which a member has a communicative disorder, issues of grief and loss are likely to emerge, disappear, re-emerge, disappear, re-emerge, etc. as the therapeutic process unfolds. According to Moses (1985), "You — the special educator, audiologist, speech-language pathologist — are the ones who deal firsthand with people who are under stress in a circumstance that is most appropriately dealt with by you rather than by psychologists, social workers, or psychiatrists. You are the people who can take a truly holistic approach in the treatment of the child within a nonpathology-oriented environment" (p. 84). We concur with this perspective and add to it our belief that this is true for clients and family members at every stage of the family life cycle, not just for families with children. When the professional uses reflective listening and responds to expressions of feeling as they occur, this normalizes the grieving and loss process and gives family members permission to be honest about their feelings and thoughts. When the clinician becomes frightened by these expressions and immediately refers to another professional because *he/she* is uncomfortable, this creates another problem for the family. They may think that there is now something else wrong with them, thereby adding to the stress they are already experiencing. In most cases when a family or family members decide to seek professional counseling, this will be a choice that they themselves initiate. The clinician should strongly support their decision. The willingness to allow expressions of feeling helps those who want additional counseling to be empowered to seek that help when they have decided that they are ready. We have never experienced a need to refer to a psychologist, social worker, or psychiatrist for counseling, but would not hesitate to do so if we were certain that it was in the best interest of our clients. Once the referral is made, it is up to the client and family to decide if they want to act on the suggestion that has been offered.

Stages of Loss

Several authors have described stages of crisis and loss by suggesting process models to consider when dealing with the emotions expressed by clients and family members who are dealing with issues of disability (Fortier and Wanlass, 1984; Moses, 1985; Spanbock, 1987). The crisis stages suggested by Fortier and Wanlass (1984) will be used here, acknowledging that other models can be equally helpful. The clinician should be familiar with crisis stages so that he/she can respond appropriately to family members. Therefore, counseling responses are described as well. The stages are impact, denial, grief, focusing outward, and closure (Fortier and Wanlass, 1984).

Impact occurs when the family and client first learn of the disability or of an accident that is likely to lead to future disability. An infant born with a bilateral cleft lip and palate, diagnosis of severe to profound hearing loss, a closed head injury, or a stroke are examples of events that trigger the impact stage. When the communicative disorder is one of the results of a life threatening accident, there may be a brief period of elation related to the relief of knowing that the loved one will not die (Spanbock, 1987). However, this elation is short-lived as reality sets in.

Occasionally, suspicion that a problem exists has been part of the family's life for several weeks, months, or years and the agonizing wait finally culminates in a diagnosis that confirms their fears. This may occur when a hearing loss is finally recognized, an infant's cerebral palsy is diagnosed, or the effects of a head injury become clearly evident. In these cases the impact stage may be prolonged, but a point is always reached where the reality of the situation impacts the family and the client. During the impact stage family members experience numbness, disorientation, nausea, agitation, muscle tension, and a number of other physically and emotionally destabilizing effects. This is certainly not a time for professional lectures or cheerful assurances that "everything is going to be just fine." Instead, the professional should present all information in it's simplest form understanding that the same information will probably have to be repeated later since not all of it will be "heard." Questions should be answered honestly, directly and simply. The clinician should allow silence and give family members an opportunity to say what they need to say. The clinician can use reflection as needed and show a calm presence that offers assurance of future assistance even as the family and client are grieving their loss.

The *denial* stage may begin soon after impact or may emerge weeks or months later. Moses (1985) reiterates that denial is necessary, healthy, and important and buys time for people to find the inner strength and the external supports to deal with the "undealable." Luterman (1984), also confirms that " . . . denial is a very normal and human reaction, which occurs in all of us" (p.150). The clinician is wise to view family denial in this same way. In addition, it is advisable to avoid "professional denial" that may occur when the clinician pretends that nothing tragic has happened and that the disability can be fully overcome. During the denial stage family members may experience tenseness, anxiety, ambivalence, disbelief, anger, avoidance, and may "shop" for cures. The clinician can use clarification, reflection and neutral questioning very effectively as the family works at figuring out the issues that they can and cannot handle. Family members are able to work on plans for change even while the denial is present. The clinician's understanding of this will be woven into the fabric of treatment.

Grief is another stage in the loss process that may also be part of the previous two stages. Grief is often expressed through crying. Anger, withdrawal, sleeplessness, guilt, self doubt, questioning and reliving the past are other common expressions associated with this stage. Again, the professional should exhibit a calm presence and allow these expressions of feeling to occur. Acknowledgment of the acceptability of grief is shown through reflection and as this is done most family members eventually dry their tears and ask to continue with the treatment process.

Focusing outward is the next stage that evolves out of the former three. Family members express relief that "the worst is over," show renewed energy and confidence, become active in considering options, and seek new knowledge and information. Other expressions of feelings may reappear during this stage, but the general tone is one of hope and fresh optimism. Persons who have been free to express the feelings felt during the impact, denial, and grief stages are likely to enter this phase with a sense of renewal in spite of the monumental challenges that lie ahead. Clarification, neutral questioning, creative strategizing, and task assignment can all be utilized by the clinician during the focusing outward stage.

Fortier and Wanlass' (1984) last stage is *closure*. At this time family members are generally calm and relaxed and have adjusted to their changed family member. The physical symptoms that were prominent earlier have diminished considerably. Family members often acknowledge, "I'm able to sleep again," or, "I can finally enjoy eating again." Continuing external support, creative strategizing, clarification, neutral questioning, and task assignment are techniques that should be used as treatment efforts proceed, sometimes on a long-term basis.

Variations in the Loss Process

An understanding of the loss process will increase the professional's sensitivity to the emotional and physical pain that often accompanies speech-language problems. Appropriate responses are woven into the fabric of treatment in a way that may be almost imperceptible to someone unfamiliar with the power of respectful and empathic listening because these responses do not dominate the treatment process. The stages and correct responses are described here to give the clinician techniques to use when the need arises. These do not supplant the clinician's primary task which is to involve the family in the treatment process. Nevertheless, additional consideration must be given to the factors described below since these relate to the grieving and loss process.

Every individual in a family will respond differently to the loss experienced and is likely to traverse the stages with different pacing and timing. For example, a father may show little emotion especially during the early phases of the process, perhaps because of his desire to remain strong in light of his wife's open expression of grief, or he may be a person who usually does not show emotion and this becomes a time when that particular personality trait is evident. Conversely, he may be very open to showing disappointment, sorrow, and anger while his partner evidences little overt expression of feelings. An individual whose life pattern has been to accept disappointment in a calm manner will continue to show that same pattern as the current distress is felt. An individual whose style is to openly express feelings will continue to respond overtly when grief and loss are experienced. Respect for these individual differences is critical and the professional is advised to refrain from "telling" people what they *should* be feeling or which stage they *should* be experiencing. The loss stages are offered as a guide for professionals who want to be sensitive to the grieving process while also respectful of individual and family differences. A polyocular view is critical to the successful treatment of families that are experiencing and expressing grief.

    The grief process is not one that is smoothly traversed and then completed. Stages repeat themselves, sorrow and pain may re-emerge at developmental transitions, and "mini" grief processes may appear for a few hours or days years after the original impact has occurred. One father told us that he had forgotten that his son, Carl, was developmentally disabled until he enrolled him in preschool and saw the other children attending the special education class. At that time he was once again reminded that Carl was not "normal." This father had evolved through the loss process to closure over a period of 13 to 14 months as he and his wife worked together to provide for and enjoy their son. As Carl approached and began his developmental transition into the pre-school years, elements of the loss process re-emerged and his parents experienced several days of renewed grief that was, however, not as intense as it had been during the early stages of the loss process. These feelings are likely to re-emerge when Carl starts elementary school, when his age cohorts begin dating and driving, when the time for adult independence arrives, and as his parents age and they and he become concerned about his lifetime care.

Finally, the loss process is experienced at every phase of the family life cycle. An aging couple whose retirement plans are changed by a debilitating stroke, a young adult whose life plans are wiped out by a severe head injury, and a young family giving up their dream of a "perfect" child all need the skills of a sensitive clinician as they and other family members work to solve the speech-language problems that are a significant part of their loss.

CONCLUSION

Counseling techniques enhance the effectiveness of the speech-language clinician during all phases of Family Based Treatment. Like the basil in a fine tomato sauce, the blue thread in a woven fabric, or the second violin in a string orchestra, these techniques become an integral part of the process and outcome of treatment. Family Based Treatment may be possible without their use but will be more satisfying, complete, and successful when these human relation skills are used by the clinician during the treatment process.

CHAPTER 10

APPLICATION TO EARLY CHILDHOOD SPEECH, LANGUAGE, HEARING PROBLEMS

Families begin, evolve, change, and endure over a span of many years. As the life span increases, families expand to three, four, and sometimes five generations of individuals who are inextricably related through intergenerational time. Each generation moves through stages that evolve from one phase to another as members enter and leave the family system. Family theorists have suggested a number of different family developmental stage models (Duvall, 1977; Haley, 1973; Solomon, 1973). The model used in this book is proposed by Carter and McGoldrick (1980). Their six stage model includes (1) the unattached young adult; (2) the joining of families through marriage; (3) the family with young children; (4) the family with adolescents; (5) launching children and moving on; and (6) the family in later life. Developmental disruptions, such as divorce, remarriage, illness, early death, or disability have a profound effect on families as they evolve through these stages. An understanding of the stages, developmental tasks, transitional stressors, and developmental disruptions that accompany the family's developmental process will enhance the clinician's use of the Family Based Treatment model. The next three chapters will identify the developmental factors that we have found to be particularly salient to speech-language treatment during different phases of the family life cycle. In this book we have divided our discussion of developmental stages into three broadened categories. Early childhood, school-age, and adulthood will be discussed as these stages relate to the treatment of specific speech-language disorders. Family variables will be emphasized, but the goal of speech-language change is always primary. We will use examples from our work with families and relate these to a variety of speech-language-hearing disorders. The cases have been sufficiently disguised to protect the identity of the families, but all are accurate examples of the content and process of our work.

FAMILY DEVELOPMENTAL FACTORS OF EARLY CHILDHOOD

Many significant changes are required of families as children enter the system. Parents adjust the marital dyad to make space for new family members, the parenting role is gradually learned, and relationships with extended family members are realigned in order to include the parental and grandparental roles (Carter & McGoldrick, 1980). While these family changes are negotiated, the married couple must also take care to attend to their relationship and the solo parent must develop and maintain adult relationships. Life becomes more complex as a newly created two generation system negotiates the paradigmatic shifts in thinking and behaving that accompany the integration of new members into the system. Nevertheless, families who enjoy a history of successful problem-solving and whose economic resources are adequate will move through the transition with a fair amount of ease. The complexity of the transition, however, may become overwhelming to families lacking in problem solving skills, living in poverty, or struggling to maintain a minimally adequate standard of living.

The New Family Member

As parents make space for children, their foreknowledge of developmental expectations is helpful but seldom fully prepares them for the advent of the new family member. Several family specialists have used the term "crisis" to describe the birth or adoption of the first child (LeMasters, 1957; Burr, 1972; Dyer, 1963). Family disruption, chronic fatigue, and the temperament of the infant are some of the factors that affect parents as they accommodate to their new family member. As the child matures and additional children join the family, new challenges confront parents as they attempt to deal with the rapidly evolving developmental milestones associated with the early childhood years. In addition, couples with young children generally report lower marital satisfaction than do couples in later stages of the family life cycle (Rollins & Feldman, 1970). These developmental issues, along with the countless joys and pleasures associated with the early childhood years, are common in families whose children are "normal." The disruption of developmental delay and disability adds significantly to the problems that must be dealt with during these early years.

When a child is born with a developmental disability or when a problem is identified during the early years, family members have to deal with the "loss of the dream" (Moses, 1985). Their dream of the perfect child, once envisioned, is destroyed and the family must begin the slow process of getting to know this "new" child. Speech-language pathologists working with families during this time will encounter parents at various stages in the loss process who are also dealing with other issues of development associated with this child as well as parenting their other children. We are continually impressed by the stamina and energy shown by these parents.

Another situation encountered by almost all families confronted with early childhood delay and disability is the plethora of differing professional opinions that parents must sort through in order to make wise decisions regarding treatment. Families have had no preparation for dealing with this complex array of advice, often presented with a certainty that is simultaneously overwhelming and confusing. The fortunate parents who feel certain about what is best for their child or who encounter a professional that is supportive of their efforts to maintain their appropriate role as decision-makers will be empowered and strengthened as they deal with the challenges and joys of parenting a young child. This sense of competence will be conveyed to the child who will, in turn, benefit from the stability offered by the self-confident parents.

Finally, as the family accommodates to its new member, the nagging uncertainty of the eventual outcome of the effects of the delay or disability may be an added stressor. As the child matures his/her potential becomes clearer, but during the early years uncertainty prevails. Some families are unable to get an exact diagnosis of the problem or may be given several different diagnoses. Even when the diagnosis is clear, the prognosis is often less certain. Family Based Treatment gives the family permission to struggle with the clinician as, together, they work to create change so that the child's full speech-language potential during the early years of development is realized.

New Couple and Parenting Roles

When a child is born into a family, the married couple has to change their way of relating to one another. When the parent is a solo parent, she/he must adapt to a significantly altered adult lifestyle while learning to parent the child alone unless grandparents, siblings, or friends are available for help and support. All through the family life cycle the importance of maintaining satisfying and enriching adult relationships is vital to the well-being of parents who, in turn, are strengthened to provide the nurturing and care that is vital to the well-being of their children. This task can be a particularly arduous one for families having a young child with special needs.

The task of maintaining the couple relationship is especially challenging when one parent is responsible for taking the child to appointments with professionals and then attempts to follow the prescribed directives of each of these professionals and translate that information to the spouse. In most two parent families mother accepts this role while father focuses his energy on work and career demands. Many mothers are forced to temporarily give up or cut back on their career plans as caregiving responsibilities become a priority. Other mothers must figure out how to meet job responsibilities while also attending to the frequent professional appointments engendered by their children's special needs. The speech-language pathologist can make a significant contribution to the well-being of families in the early childhood years by arranging appointments at times that are convenient to both parents. Fathers are willing participants when it is clear that their involvement is useful and wanted. We have never had a father in a two parent family turn down our invitation to participate in treatment. Our efforts to enlist fathers on the treatment team have paid off in benefits to their children, enrichment of our treatment planning, and cohesiveness of the family as the couple engages in mutual decision-making relative to their child.

If the child lives in a solo parent family and if the custodial parent agrees, we always ask the child's non-custodial parent to join the treatment team. An affirmative response is usually received. Parents, of course, can divorce one another but can never divorce their children and usually want to remain active in the child's life. We also like to include grandparents, aunts, uncles, live-in friends, and other supportive individuals who are available to assist the solo parent and/or who may have direct influence on the treatment of the communicative disorder. These individuals can, at the parents' request, act as co-parents with the busy mother of a preschooler and offer valuable support as the speech-language disorder is treated.

Sometimes professionals become overzealous in their desire to promote change and expect parents to provide almost constant reinforcement and stimulation to their children. Instead, clinicians should be sensitive to potential parental exhaustion and can suggest that it might be best for the child if the parents took a night out or arranged for time together and focused on their own adult interests. This time "away" can help parents refuel and develop renewed energy for the challenges presented by a child with special needs.

Finally, we want to urge clinicians to support parents

in their appropriate role thus empowering parents to make decisions about their children. These decisions will not always be the same as those the professional would like parents to make, but unless the clinician plans to be responsible for the child until the child reaches maturity or is no longer in need of services, that right is the parents' alone. We must take great care to avoid usurping the parental role. Instead, it is more appropriate to support and enhance the interactive resources that parents bring to treatment.

The Extended Family

When a first child is born, parents are also "born." In many cases, grandparents are also created for the first time. Even if the couple has had few expressed differences prior to the birth of the child differences are very likely to emerge at this point. Each parent was parented by different people, and grandparental opinions often become a significant part of the family system at this point. When parents are confident, supportive of one another, able to deal with differences, and can enlist the grandparents as *consultants* to the parenting process, the transition will be fairly smooth. Extended family conflict can erupt, however, if grandparents become uninvited experts who disqualify the fledgling parents as they are learning their new role. Such conflict, if not resolved after the birth of the first child, continues both overtly and covertly with the birth of subsequent children. Again, the introduction of new grandparents, great grandparents, aunts, and uncles into a family can be a stressful process when the child shows no unusual problems. When developmental delay or disability is evident, the differences between the parents themselves and between parents, grandparents, and other significant family members is often heightened.

Extended family members are important additions to the treatment team when their presence is desired by the parent or parents. When the parent is a solo parent, grandparents and great-grandparents often have frequent contact with the child and are able to offer significant assistance as strategies for change are identified. All decisions, however, must be finally approved by the parent so that her role as the primary caregiver of her child is strengthened. Ordinarily, we begin treatment with the child and parent alone unless they are living in the grandparental home. When the grandparents have knowledge, resources, and influence that can be accessed for speech-language change, it is a good idea to enlist their participation in the decision-making process.

When intergenerational differences in two parent families appear to be focused on problems related to speech-language difficulties, we work with the parents to plan a three generational meeting in which the goals of treatment are described and the grandparents' resources are identified. The act of convening this large group of people, all of whom love and care for the child in question, usually eases the intergenerational conflict and produces new ideas for change.

Finally, in most cases, the three or four generations of each family are already joined in their concern for the well-being of the child with a communicative disorder even before the speech-language pathologist enlists their support. When this reciprocal love and concern is accessed and recognized, possibilities for change are expanded and the child benefits greatly.

EARLY CHILDHOOD CASE STUDIES

Language Development

According to Snow (1984) there have been two major changes over the past twenty years in the way we think about the development of language. First, we have shifted our emphasis from language to communication; second, the mother-child dyad has replaced the child alone as the unit of study. These changes are not only true for research in language development but are evident in the treatment of language learning disorders. Within the past five years clinical emphasis has expanded from the mother-child dyad to the family, and clinicians are writing Individual Family Service Plans (Johnson et al., 1989).

Clearly, not all parents who request an assessment of their child's communicative ability believe that there is a problem nor do two parents necessarily agree on whether or not a problem exists. In a surprising number of instances, parents have met with us in order to satisfy grandparents, preschool screeners, or a professional person who believed that a problem existed. In other cases, one or both parents were extremely concerned and attempts to elicit speech and language were failing. For these reasons, it is very important to learn the point of view of each family member early in the first session, to discuss agreement or disagreement between parents, and to compare and contrast the parents views with those of anyone outside the immediate family who believes that a problem may exist. While it is possible to conduct an assessment without this information, it is not possible to offer the same quality of service as that provided by the clinician who has this information and uses it to find points of accommodation and to assist parents in developing a clearer definition of their own perspective.

Mark was nearly three years old and ignored his parents' efforts to encourage him to say words. His mother was very concerned; his father was not. Mark's maternal grandmother was most concerned and encouraged her adult daughter to pursue treatment for Mark even if his father "didn't care." Margo, Mark's mother, read about screening services for young children that were available in the community and decided that this might be a good way to find out if Mark did, indeed, have a problem. At the screening assessment Margo was told that Mark was delayed in language development and she was asked to return for a second follow-up appointment. Margo and Al, together, took Mark for the second appointment. Only later did we learn of Al's anger in response to a comment made by one of the testers during the assessment to the effect that parents nowadays were fortunate because placement was available up to age twenty-one

Application to Early Childhood

no matter how delayed a child was.

It was shortly after that assessment that we met Mark, his parents, and his eight-year-old sister. During that first session, neither Mark nor his father spoke much. On the other hand, mother and daughter talked animatedly, each interrupting and "talking over" the other. Margo was clearly the spokesperson of the family and she was first to describe Mark's lack of talking and some of the things she had done to help him. These included looking at books with him and asking him to imitate words she said. She cried occasionally as she described her concern about Mark's lack of communication. Al was very quiet throughout the session, but indicated that he too had been slow to talk and that Mark, like him, would talk when he was ready and wanted to. Rachael, Mark's sister, indicated that she liked to help Mark and did so by asking him to imitate words that she said. The counseling techniques of clarifying, reflecting, and summarizing were used to learn the parents' views of the problem, to respond to Margo's emotions, and to encourage participation in treatment. After listening to the views of all family members, we summarized the view of each parent as we understood it and found a point of accommodation for the parents' differing opinions as to whether or not Mark had a communicative problem: "Al, you think that Mark is *able* to talk, but like you've been told that you were at his age, he just isn't interested or ready for some unknown but perhaps familial reason. You really become angry when teachers or other school personnel suggest that he might be retarded because you find him to be pretty smart when it comes to tools and doing mechanical things with his hands. Margo, you on the other hand, are very worried and have been looking at books with Mark and asking him to imitate words you say in order to help him, but so far these things sometimes result in Mark saying a word but often not. Al, if we find that we agree with Margo....that is, that we think that Mark could benefit from us working together to help him, would you be willing to participate in order to support Margo and her concern?" As has often occurred in similar families we have seen, framing Al's participation in services as being for the purpose of supporting his wife enlisted his cooperation. Initially disinterested since he believed that no problem existed, he became actively involved since he was now doing something for his wife.

By this time we were beginning to feel joined with the family. Al became more talkative immediately after we acknowledged his belief that Mark did not have a problem. He talked about how concerned Margo was and acknowledged that even he sometimes wondered when Mark would talk. We discussed in detail the things that Mark's family members did to help him and observed, as we talked, the interactions that were enacted between Mark and members of his family. Mark, for example, played with a soccer ball by holding it and tracing the lines on the ball with his finger. His sister talked to him a lot in a seeming effort to get his attention, but Mark seldom responded. When she hit the ball out of his hand, he showed no signs of objection but picked up a puzzle piece from the floor and began examining it. Margo described Mark's interest in books and how Mark seemed to like that activity sometimes but not at others. Tracking was used to learn what happened when he "enjoyed" looking at books with her and what usually happened when he did not. When we asked Al what he did to help Mark, he responded that he liked to wrestle on the floor with him, watch television with him, and go for rides with him in an old car that he had restored.

After learning about the parents' view of the problem, listening for agreements and disagreements, finding points of accommodation when appropriate, listening for mobilization points, and watching enactments, we asked Margo to look at a book with Mark as we watched. Mark sat on Margo's lap and Margo typically pointed to pictures as she asked Mark, "What's this?" Mark looked at the first three or four pictures to which his mother pointed. He did not say the word in response to her question. On one occasion, Margo named the picture as she pointed, "Here's a car," and Mark looked. He did not phonate or verbally respond in any noticeable way. Soon Rachael joined her mother and began asking Mark questions about the pictures also. After about two minutes, Al asked Rachael to come and sit with him which she did.

Several resources became evident in this three or four minute enactment. First, although it was difficult to obtain a shared focus of attention with Mark, he looked at the first several pictures that his mother showed him. Second, his mother liked to look at books with him and encouraged Mark to name pictures. Third, Mark's sister was interested in helping her mother help Mark. Fourth, Al helped his wife by asking Rachael to come and sit with him. Fifth, Rachael responded to her father's request which was an indication that the parents were appropriately in charge of the children. These were resources that could be amplified, expanded, and made more effective. By capitalizing on these we would be able to give an isomorphic assignment, one that fit with activities in which the family was already engaged. Other potential resources which we wanted to keep in mind for further exploration were Al's playful wrestling with Mark, Al's taking Mark for rides in the antique car, and Rachael's enjoyment of playing with Mark.

At that point we asked the parents to play with Mark using some blocks and toy animals. Mark picked up one of the animals and examined it as his parents showed him other animals and asked him what the names of the animals were. Mark neither answered their questions nor looked at them as they attempted to interact with him. Gradually the clinician joined the parents and Mark playing on the floor and began experimenting with different ways of interacting with Mark in an effort to increase visual contact, to establish one or more joint focuses of attention, and to elicit words and appropriate behavioral responses from Mark. As the clinician interacted with Mark, both parents stopped talking and watched. When the clinician reduced the amount of verbal input and quietly named the toy horse and held it so Mark could clearly see it, Mark looked. The clinician gently patted him on the back and quietly reinforced Mark verbally. When the clinician said nothing but put the horse on one of the blocks, Mark looked again as if to see what was happening. The clinician pointed to the horse again but said nothing. Mark continued to watch.

This type of play continued as the clinician experimented, with the parents sitting on the floor next to him, in search of the best interactive behavior which could be elicited from Mark. The techniques of naming objects rather than asking Mark to name them, reducing verbal input, sitting physically close to Mark, reinforcing Mark with physical contact and quiet words, pointing to objects, and limiting the number of toys available at any one time seemed to be useful in gaining Mark's attention. Mark did not say any words during the evaluation, but did phonate quietly once or twice during that ten minutes of interaction. The clinician reinforced that behavior. Once again, the parents were also sitting on the floor and watching closely as the clinician interacted with their son. They were a part of the interaction even though they said little or nothing. Their presence, as well as that of Mark's sister, was significant not only because they all observed some techniques different from what they had tried previously, but because they gave entree' to Mark. It is very likely that Mark's cooperation was due in part to the comfort he felt in the presence of his family.

One of the goals of the first session was to determine the best interactive behavior in which Mark engaged and the circumstances surrounding it. After the first fifty minutes it seemed that it was difficult for

Mark's parents and sister to engage Mark in interactive behavior. He did, however, look at several pictures in a book with his mother when she pointed to them. He also responded well when the amount of verbal input was reduced and when he was not asked questions. We discussed the positive way in which Mark responded to his mother when they first started looking at the book and when we played with the toy animals and blocks with him.

As the hour was drawing to a close, we suggested that we would like to interact more with Mark at our next session to learn more, if the parents wished to continue meeting, and that we would discuss goals at that session. Both parents agreed that they would like to return for further sessions. We discussed the mobilization points and family resources and complimented Margo for looking at books with Mark and for her recognition of the importance of that activity. We complimented both parents for their gentle firmness with their children and said that we noticed how well Rachael responded when Al asked her to sit with him. We also complimented Rachael for playing nicely with Mark as we talked and especially for listening to Mark and sometimes not talking so that Mark could say words and make sounds if he wanted to. We delivered the following assignments:

1. Notice the times that Mark looks at you and when you feel "linked" with him. Pay attention to those situations and make notes about them to bring next time.

2. Margo, look at books with Mark at times when you believe that he will be interested. As you do so, you name the pictures and point to them, but don't ask Mark to say anything. Pay attention to his responses, but try not to ask him any questions or ask him to name any of the pictures during those times.

3. Al, pay particular attention to what you do and to what Mark does when you two are "wrestling." Notice how much you talk, the extent to which Mark makes sounds, whether or not Mark imitates any "grunts" and "groans" you make, the extent to which he looks at you, whether or not he does things to you to which he expects a response, etc. We'll talk about what you noticed next week and even have you show us what you do.

4. Rachael, we liked the way you played with Mark. We especially liked the way you were quiet sometimes to let Mark talk if he wanted to. This week, as you play with him try hard to remember to listen carefully for any words that Mark says or sounds that he makes.

5. Please call the office to make an appointment for a hearing test for Mark just to rule this out as a factor.

We discussed the assignment to be sure that everyone understood it and agreed to meet in one week.

The second session began with a discussion of the assignment. Both parents were more keenly aware of the difficulty they had in obtaining Mark's attention and interacting with him visually and also of techniques for improving that aspect of Mark's interactive behavior. Al described the situation as being "pretty bad when you're ignored by a three year old" and indicated that he understood better what Margo was concerned about. Both parents had noticed that Mark looked at them when he pointed to the cupboard requesting dry cereal to eat with his fingers. We tracked that event and found that not only did Mark look at the parent but that he said an approximation of the brand name of the cereal. When asked what

Margo and Al did in response, both indicated that they gave him the box of cereal. When we asked specifically if they repeated the word Mark had approximated or showed pleasure that he had said a word both, parents said that they merely gave him the cereal. We suggested that they use that opportunity to let Mark know how pleased they were and to say the word back to him several times.

We asked Margo and Al what happened when they tried making written notes about Mark's attentiveness. Both indicated that they had forgotten to do that. We discussed the feasibility of writing notes and both agreed that it would be very difficult for them to take time to do that. They added that paper and pencils were not sitting out in their home. We agreed that this was not a part of the assignment that fit their lifestyle and commended them for remembering the events so well.

Margo reported that looking at the books had gone well and that Mark seemed especially interested in them when she named the pictures rather than asking him to do so. However, she expressed concern because Mark did not say the names and felt that this was, therefore, not helping him. When we tracked exactly what had happened, Margo described how on several occasions Mark had pointed to a picture after she named it. We told her that we thought that this was real progress and that she had done a good job. We discussed communicative development with Margo and Al and emphasized the importance of social interaction and listening as a part of that. Both seemed satisfied. We did not point out that asking Mark questions and telling him to say words had not elicited words either. We could have given a noticing assignment had the parents continued to be concerned about what we viewed as progress.

We discussed Al's wrestling assignment and Al had noticed that wrestling elicited a lot of responses from Mark. Mark not only had looked at him, but also tickled Al and waited for a response. Al noticed that Mark imitated noises that Al made and reported that he had repeated these again in response to Mark's imitation. We discussed how this could lead to words that Mark might naturally imitate and decided that this should be built into the next assignment. As we talked about Al and Mark wrestling, Mark looked at us and seemed to be monitoring our conversation as he played with toys with Rachael. Because Mark, at that moment, was playing purposely with the toys, we called it to Al and Margo's attention and discussed how different that type of play looked as opposed to tracing the lines on the soccer ball which we had observed Mark do the previous week. Eventually Al and Mark did put on their "wrestling exhibition" for us and we commented on the many good features that we saw mentioning particularly those that Al had noticed at home as we saw them enacted during the session. Al grunted and groaned and Mark imitated him readily. Al said a word, but Mark did not respond. Nevertheless, this clearly was a resource upon which we could expand.

We met with Mark and his family fourteen more times during the next six months. The results of the hearing test showed normal hearing sensitivity. Mark continued to become increasingly responsive and began saying words and short phrases. No formal language tests were administered, but spontaneous language samples were collected periodically as Mark began using words and we attended to the purposes for which Mark used words and expanded upon these. Everyone observed Mark use language for the purpose of greeting others, to regulate the behavior of others, to exchange information, and to express feelings (Carrow-Woolfolk & Lynch, 1982). He still did not talk as readily or as much as many children his age, but his use of morphological markers was developing and he became considerably more responsive to others and more "available" for learning. Assignments were con-

Application to Early Childhood

tinued using the same type of approach used during the first session - looking for the best communicative behaviors we could elicit from Mark and building upon these, identifying and building upon family resources, combining our knowledge with the expertise and ability of the family members, and giving assignments which were both isomorphic and derived from a polyocular perspective.

Mark began attending preschool at the time of our fourteenth session and we began the transition process of linking Mark and his family with personnel from the preschool. The speech-language pathologist from the preschool attended the fifteenth session with us and observed Mark interacting with his family members. We attended the preschool staffing and acknowledged that the progress that Mark had made during the past six months was related to the expertise of his family and their concern for Mark. We encouraged Margo and Al to describe some of their activities that worked best and assumed that the teacher and speech-language pathologist would want to continue using the resources of Mark's family. Both the teacher and speech-language pathologist responded to Al and Margo by praising them for their concern and ability to help Mark. They indicated that they would like for them to continue giving input and expanding upon the activities of the preschool. We agreed that our role would be to meet once each month for the remainder of the school year and determine the need for summer services at that time. Al and Margo agreed that primary speech-language services should be offered by the speech-language pathologist at the preschool. Further, they felt confident that they knew what to do to facilitate Mark's language development at home and were ready for Mark to receive services in the context of the school. We did not schedule services for the summer because Al and Margo planned to be away much of the time. We stopped seeing them regularly that fall, but on several occasions Margo sent us a videotape of Mark interacting with her and Al, and we had a telephone conversation about their interactive techniques and Mark's responses. At last contact, Mark was enrolled in a regular kindergarten and received speech-language services in that context.

Communicative Disorders Associated With Cleft Lip/Palate

Parents, siblings, grandparents, and other relatives of a child born with a cleft lip and/or palate or any craniofacial anomaly are confronted with the physical evidence of the problem on the day of birth. The joyful preparation, excitement, tension, physical pain, and tremendous relief associated with childbirth are suddenly obliterated by shock, grief, fear, and an overwhelming sorrow. Professionals and family members wanting to console the grieving parents often make the mistake of downplaying the tragedy assuring them that surgery will correct nature's error and that things are not really so bad. Even worse, these people may tiptoe around the issue speaking in hushed tones trying to protect the exhausted mother from the reality of the situation by avoiding discussion of the event. Others may tell the parents how they "should" respond thus further negating the right of the parents to express their grief in an idiosyncratic manner. One mother of a child born with a cleft palate told us that a hospital professional had admonished her that she was not grieving properly because no one had seen her cry since the birth of her daughter. This statement further compounded her grief and left her with feelings of hurt and anger toward the insensitive professional.

More fortunate families are offered the opportunity to interact with professionals who quietly attend to their needs as the numbness subsides; who allow them to express their grief, anger, and pain; and who answer all questions honestly and simply as they arise. From the beginning of their child's life, these families are encouraged to be active participants as decisions are made. The well-being of the child is related to the well-being of the parents, and specialists in cleft palate emphasize the importance of the professional's willingness to work with family members as treatment plans are developed for the young child with a cleft lip and/or palate (Goetz, 1982; Hahn, 1979; Schwartz, 1982). These families are beginning the process of empowerment that will enable them to trust their own abilities and feelings as they face the difficult days ahead.

Michael's mother describes her reaction to the array of services and decisions that confronted her during her first months and early years with her son:

"When my child was born, I had no knowledge of the extensive treatment that was involved in his medical care. There were surgeries, orthodontics, speech therapy, ear problems and emotional development to consider. I had to rely mainly on each specialist to provide me with the necessary information needed for his growth. What I encountered was a mixture of 'professional egotism' from some of the specialists and a genuine concern for Michael's wellbeing from others.

"Michael's surgeon insisted that he be seen by a clinic that could provide a 'Team Approach.' After attending the first clinic I was told that an evaluation would be sent to me of each professional's opinion. When I read the report, I didn't understand it. It was written by professionals for professionals. When I tried to have the report explained to me, some of the specialists told me to just keep bringing him for the evaluations and they would take care of it. They knew how to treat a cleft palate child. They had worked with 6000 before. The problem was that I didn't know how or what they were treating him for. Was it possible for me to enhance areas of his development? Would I do something to retard his development? I had no way of knowing. I sought second and sometimes third opinions to become more knowledgeable of options available to my child.

"When Michael was about to begin speech therapy I heard of a clinic that incorporated the family in the treatment. It was explained to me that therapy would be

enhanced if the family members understood objectives and could help the child in his speech development. The results have been astounding. We, the professionals, the parent, and the child, as a team, have been able to accomplish goals necessary for Michael's well-being.

> "Though the results of his speech have been positive, not all other aspects are. I still find it a struggle to be incorporated in other areas of his care. There are choices, and as a parent I want to make competent decisions concerning my son's treatment. It is important to remember that each child is an individual and not just another case to be handled. The parent is as necessary as each specialist in overall treatment. Without the two working together, the child ultimately suffers, and the professional's knowledge has been of no use." (Seibel, 1987a, p.1-2)

Michael's mother, Nancy, contacted the clinician when Michael was 20 months old. She was a veteran visitor to specialists but was tentatively enthusiastic about the possibility of being more involved in the decision-making process. Her considerable energy and strong desire to remain in charge of decisions relating to her son were viewed by the clinician as assets. She and Michael's father had divorced a year earlier. Since that time Michael had almost no contact with his father, and apparently no child support was forthcoming. Our suggestion that father be included in the sessions was not supported by Nancy and her wishes were respected since she was the custodial parent. Mother and son were living with the maternal grandparents and also in close proximity to the maternal great-grandmother. This excellent support system benefited Michael since he was surrounded by many loving adults. Both grandmothers, as well as Nancy's brother, participated in sessions when Nancy felt that this was appropriate.

Michael, a blond, shy toddler was born with a complete bilateral cleft lip and palate. The cleft lip and palate had been surgically repaired although scarring in the area of the lip was clearly evident. Michael, clearly wary of another "Doctor," observed most of the first session from a safe corner of the room responding with tears when interaction with the clinician was requested. Michael's normal fears were respected and most of the first session focused on data gathering as Nancy described the speech and language characteristics that she had noticed, as well as her hopes for her son's development. Toward the end of the session, Michael approached his mother, and she was able to elicit from him some of the speech responses necessary for a beginning assessment of the problem.

As the beginning phase of treatment evolved, Michael's shyness disappeared and a bright, assertive toddler emerged. The primary goal was for Michael to develop an oral air stream for speech and to make full use of his velopharyngeal mechanism. If surgery had given him an adequate mechanism, he would learn to use it. If the mechanism was inadequate, that would become increasingly apparent. Secondary goals were to facilitate further language development and to increase mobility of the upper lip. Nancy was actively involved in a number of activities designed to meet these goals. Helping Michael increase the variety of consonant sounds by letting him watch her face and touch her lips while she blew, said babababa, papapapa, etc. and made other noises are examples of beginning procedures. Weekly sessions were held, and at each session goals and procedures were altered and changed to fit Nancy and Michael's interactive style and to elicit speech-language change. Michael's language development improved significantly. Changes in speech continued to be characterized by hypernasality and nasal air emission but Michael's considerable effort and Nancy's continuing work with him at home produced gradual speech changes.

As Michael matured and became more verbal, Nancy became very expert in her ability to reinforce his appropriate speech utterances and sessions were spaced farther apart since her use of reinforcement in the natural context was providing the stimulation that he needed. The clinician believed that a surgical reevaluation was necessary because all best efforts did not seem to bring the mechanism to its desired functioning for speech purposes. A meeting with the surgeon and Nancy was held and the decision was made to delay work on the velopharyngeal mechanism until cosmetic revision of Michael's lip was completed. This cosmetic surgery was then performed necessitating a vacation from speech-language treatment and altering the amount of effort that young Michael could muster for articulatory practice.

Following the "vacation," Family Based Treatment resumed and Michael's articulatory competence continued to improve. This competence, however, was not at a level believed appropriate and surgery was scheduled to construct and place a pharyngeal flap. Meanwhile, an orthodontic evaluation was conducted and plans were made to begin orthodontia when the flap was in place. Throughout all of these changes, speech-language treatment had to be suspended as medical and dental treatment was implemented. Nancy, however, knowledgeable in all areas of speech change, continued to help Michael when it was clear to her that he was physically able to be involved in attention to speech. Michael had evolved into a bright, intelligent, perceptive three year old who was comfortable with himself in spite of the difficulties that he endured.

As these changes occurred, Michael also was enrolled in preschool and Nancy returned to work, at first part-time and then on a full-time basis. She and Michael moved to an apartment of their own while grandmother and great-grandmother continued to assist with child care when Nancy's work schedule required such assistance. Michael began developing friendships, and Nancy was finally able to schedule

Application to Early Childhood

some personal recreation time into her life. A "normal" life style began to emerge. Meanwhile, speech-language services were maintained through monthly visits. During these sessions Nancy would report and demonstrate the interactive speech-language techniques that she was using and the clinician would then suggest new procedures as needed.

When Michael entered kindergarten, Nancy decided that he should continue speech-language treatment at school and contact was made with the speech-language clinician to share the work that had been done and to encourage the inclusion of Michael's mother in the treatment process at school. Nancy's confident, competent parenting as well as her thorough knowledge of Michael's speech-language needs and velopharyngeal capabilities empowered her to continue to make the necessary decisions associated with her maturing son. Again the reader is privileged to share Nancy's experience as she describes her personal responses to these early years with Michael.

"As an expectant parent, I was filled with feelings of excitement, anticipation and joy. I was going to be a mother. Will it be a boy or girl? What will we name it? Who will it look like? What a happy time this was and what a tremendous disappointment when I found out he was born less than perfect.

"When the doctor told me that my baby had been born with a bilateral cleft lip and palate, I felt absolutely devastated to see him so severely deformed. I couldn't believe that this had happened to me. Why was God punishing me? I had always heard that there was an immediate bond between a mother and her child. This simply wasn't the case for me, I felt no love for this baby, I felt nothing.

"After I returned to my room, people would call me and tell me to thank God it wasn't a heart defect or some other problem. However, that was no consolation to me.

You can't see a heart defect, but you could see his facial disfigurement. No one ever congratulated me on his birth. When my husband saw him, he said, "Oh, it's no big deal." My God what was he saying? Was I the only one feeling devastated, shocked and scared? How could I possibly cope?

"The surgeon came in and told me Michael would never look "normal," never like you and me, but a repair would be done. Oh, my God, this won't go away will it? What am I going to do? He told me that baby must weigh ten pounds before the closure could be done. 'Go home and enjoy your son.' How could I possibly do that? How could I possibly enjoy this baby? How could I possibly love this child? Throughout my hospital stay my husband only came up once.

"When I brought Michael home, I wasn't sure I could care for him; I wasn't sure I wanted to. As I went through the motions, I began to notice what pretty blue eyes he had, his beautiful strawberry blonde hair, and then I saw him smile. Michael was real; he was alive, and I was hurting deeply.

"At two months, Michael was ready for his first surgery, and so was I. After waiting for three hours, the surgeon came out very excited with the results. He quickly brought me to the recovery room to show me. What I saw was my baby with a lip. He was crying and had several stitches. They brought him to his room and asked me to hold him. I was scared. I didn't know how to care for him. The nurses helped me, and I did fine. My husband never came to see him. When the swelling went down and sutures removed, I had his first picture taken.

"In the next few months, I began to really enjoy Michael. He started to crawl, then walk and eventually he said 'Mama.' I never thought I could be so excited However, the excitement was mixed with fear. My husband and I divorced. Would I be able to care for Michael and myself

financially and emotionally? I knew I would do my best.

"Michael had his fourth surgery at 2 1/2 years of age. *The first night was always the hardest, but when Michael woke up and was crying, 'No more Mommy, no more. I promise I will be a good boy,' I hated myself for putting him through an elective cosmetic surgery. Why did I still care what he looked like? I loved him or thought I did. I looked out the window of the hospital and wanted to jump. I can't do it anymore. I couldn't bear to know that he thought I would be punishing him. I honestly did love him. I sought professional help for my emotional well-being and for his.*

"*In the past five years, I have learned to deal with the added pressures of a special child. I have found that I love Michael for who he is and not just for what he looks like, and in turn he loves me for those same reasons. It has not been easy, and I am sure I will continue to have difficult times, but now I know that God gave me a son that is absolutely everything that I could have asked for and more. I realize God gave me the perfect child, and I am capable of a love that I never knew existed."* (Seibel, 1987b)

Nancy's eloquent sharing of her personal journey, not yet completed, reminds each of us of our professional responsibility to attend to the feelings, needs, and parenting potential of the mothers of our preschool clients.

Stuttering

We view Family Based Treatment as a refinement of traditional treatment of early stuttering since the home environment and family interactions have received attention for many years (Van Riper, 1954). Typically mothers meet with the speech-language pathologist, and fathers and siblings are not involved in treatment. Further, family interactions may be described as they are experienced by the mother, but since the rest of the family is not present, interactions are seldom observed and the perspectives of other family members are not heard. Family Based Treatment expands the treatment possibilities since the speech-language pathologist has the benefit of a polyocular view, has access to family resources, directly observes family interactions, and tracks other interactive events.

As the speech-language pathologist joins the family system and participates in the family's interactions, the clinician may sense and be affected by the emotions or feelings of family members. The same pressures, playfulness, anxiety, defensiveness, elation, depression, etc. felt by family members is often felt by the clinician. This is especially useful in cases of early stuttering because it gives the clinician additional, although very subjective, information about what the child may be experiencing. When there is tension between parents, pressure on a child to "be correct" or to react in particular preset structured ways, competition between family members, etc. the child is likely to sense this. Just as it is not uncommon for the clinician to feel this to the point that his/her own participation in interactions are tempered in order to be "appropriate," the child is likely doing the same thing but at a more rudimentary level. The ways in which these feelings and attitudes are manifested in family interactions may be the critical point. For example, when the content of parent-child play is limited to opportunities to educate the child and the interactions of play consist primarily of asking the child questions or telling him/her facts, the child who is experiencing early stuttering may feel pressure just as the clinician who attempts to play with the child "in the correct way" will feel pressure. The climate of interaction in such a case may be a variable which could be changed and manipulated in an effort to influence fluency.

We also suggest that the *normal* parental conflict experienced by parents during the early years may affect the child who is predisposed to early stuttering. This conflict can affect the parents' ability to provide consistent structure for the child. The child, in turn, may become confused and agitated thus creating a situation that is not conducive to effective communication. Access to such interactions and accommodation of parental differences may influence fluency modification efforts.

Kyle was nearly four years old and had repetitions of sounds and syllables on about five to ten percent of his words. Tension in muscles of his neck accompanied some of his disfluencies. His family consisted of his mother, the family spokesperson; his father, who had himself received treatment for stuttering and articulation as a child; and his seven year old brother, a bright and articulate child who seemed to know every detail of the family's life and was frequently called upon by his parents to remind them about past family events, incidences, places, dates, etc. Kyle's brother was a veritable encyclopedia who not only remembered these data but excelled in school with little or no effort.

Kyle was referred in the late spring by his preschool speech-language pathologist who had been seeing him for both numerous articulation errors and disfluencies. We agreed that we would see Kyle and his family over the summer, if they were interested, and focus particularly on the disfluencies since they were of increasing concern to his parents. The family was convened shortly after the referral. The preschool speech-language pathologist was not present though it would have been a good idea to ask the parents if they would have liked for her to be included at the first session.

Conversation in Kyle's family was frequent and fast-paced. Kyle's mother talked a lot. During the first session the only pressure felt by the clinician was that he had to work very hard to participate as a speaker rather than strictly a listener. Kyle's brother talked a lot, too, and he and Kyle played together during a good part of the first session. Kyle showed little indication of monitoring our conversation, but his brother was obviously doing so and sometimes corrected his parents about the details of family events they described. Kyle's father spoke infrequently. Both he and Kyle often had their conversational turns usurped or cut short by someone interrupting them. Still, the clinician felt comfortable interacting with the family and the parents seemed accepting of both boys. No particular stress or tension was apparent even though conversational "space" was limited due to the mother's ability to talk in an animated and fast-paced manner.

Consistent with the high value placed on conversation, the family did not own a television set. They valued education and self development highly; both parents were professors. Both showed acceptance of Kyle and talked about his assets which included being a relaxed and comfortable child. Family members enjoyed his company. Both parents were concerned about Kyle's fluency, but both also felt that he would likely become more fluent since that had been the father's experience. Both parents likened Kyle to his father and Kyle's brother to his mother.

Family resources evident at the first session included the fact that the family enjoyed playing games together, that both boys liked to read or be read to and that this occurred nearly every evening. Also, Kyle was "easy going" and seldom became upset, Kyle's brother liked to play with him and was generally helpful by nature, and the parents self-reported that mother talked a lot. They agreed that they both talked fast even though they thought that perhaps they should try to speak more slowly.

During the first session, the clinician played a game of checkers with Kyle and spoke very little. All of the clinician's talking was at a reduced though natural rate. He paid particular attention to allowing pause time after Kyle had spoken. Both parents and Kyle's brother watched the game. At one time or another, all gave Kyle advice; the clinician did not respond to this. The room was noticeably quiet during the game, particularly in contrast to the previous thirty minutes when the parents were being interviewed. After the game the adults discussed what had occurred, and both parents expressed surprise that an adult could play with a child and keep the child's interest without talking most of the time. This idea formed the basis for the first assignment which was isomorphic to the parents' expression that they should probably slow the rate of their own speech. It was polyocular in that they had experienced a new way of interacting with a child which included a slow, conversational rate with reduced verbal output and an absence of questions. The assignment was systemic in that a slower rate of speech was to be incorporated into natural interactions with Kyle. The specific assignment was:

> For about fifteen minutes each day, try to speak slowly when interacting with Kyle. As you suggested, this could be done when you are looking at books with him. Modify the length of time up or down to fit your schedule and notice:
>
> 1. Is this possible to do?
>
> 2. What is the effect on Kyle's speech? (eg., Did he slow his rate, too? Were disfluencies evident? Did he talk more? Less? etc.)

Subsequent sessions consisted of an elaboration of this theme of rate of speech and pause-time, use of questions by the parents, and attention to turn-taking interactions. Techniques for maintaining Kyle's feeling of self-worth in relation to his brother were discussed and other variables possibly related to periods of disfluency were examined. Kyle's parents were rewarded for their insights into Kyle's disfluency and for their ability to notice potential fluency disrupters. Isomorphic, polyocular, and systemic assignments were carried out by the family.

Predictably, Kyle's fluency varied over the ten month period. One week when Kyle had been ill and was still weak, his disfluencies were especially severe. At the same time, his family noticed that they did have influence over other situations that seemed related to disfluency. They noticed that when they stopped interrupting Kyle and gave him plenty of time to complete his conversational turn, when they rewarded his efforts to be appropriately in charge or in control of his life, and when they reduced the number of questions they asked him his fluency improved. Other effective techniques included reducing their own amount of talking and their requests for Kyle to talk during periods of disfluency, ignoring some of Kyle's articulation errors rather than attempting to correct them, and preparing Kyle for anticipated changes in routine.

Kyle and his family were seen each week during the summer for six one-hour sessions. We continued to work with them for an additional ten sessions after school began in the fall. These ten sessions were spread over an eight month period. In all, the family was seen by us for seventeen one-hour sessions over a period of eleven months. He also received treatment at school from the speech-language pathologist when school resumed in the fall. While our primary focus of concern, by mutual agreement, was fluency, at school the clinician's focus of concern was articulation and speech intelligibility. This was a general guideline, however, and we each monitored both communicative behaviors and could not help but overlap occasionally in our efforts. Treatment with us was terminated at the seventeenth session by mutual agreement. Kyle's parents had heard no stuttering for over a month and felt that they were capable of controlling the stuttering through adjusting the environment if the disfluencies returned. The speech-language pathologist at Kyle's school agreed and continued to work with Kyle on articulation. This provided an opportunity for another person to monitor Kyle's fluency. Three years post-treatment, Kyle was a fluent and intelligible speaker and a slightly above-average student. His parents enjoyed the satisfaction of having helped their own child, and it seemed that their feelings of competence would likely generalize to other inevitable and normal problem situations that would arise before Kyle reached adulthood.

Hearing Impairment

Parents of young children with hearing impairments experience varying amounts of stress related to the severity of the loss, the hearing status of the parents, the availability of services, and the family's ability to solve problems. Confusion created by the various communication options available and the conflicting advice offered by concerned extended family members and professional helpers is an additional stressor. The speech-language pathologist should always include the parents, siblings, and in many cases grandparents in the treatment process of young deaf children. Parents then have the opportunity to learn about communication options and choose those that will be most functional for them (Moores, 1985; Northern & Downs, 1974). In addition, the parents' active involvement in treatment serves to alleviate some of their stress as their energy is directed toward helping their child in a meaningful way.

The communicative environment of the child is greatly enriched when the significant others in the child's everyday context struggle with the clinician to choose, develop, implement, and reinforce strategies that lead to communicative competence. This participation empowers parents to be actively involved in the decision-making process. The sense of mastery, competence, and autonomy that is engendered is then conveyed to the child who also learns to master the environment in a developmentally appropriate manner (Schlesinger, 1985). When family members are excluded, the child is further isolated from the people who have the most potential to nurture, love and communicate with her/him.

Jennifer was the first child born to her hearing parents, Paula and Steve Miller. The family's initial contact with the speech-language pathologist was when Jennifer was two years, six months old. Historical information was gradually revealed as treatment progressed.

Paula's pregnancy, labor, and delivery were uneventful. She returned to work following a three month leave of absence from her secretarial position. Steve, a computer programmer, commuted one hour each way to his job with a large accounting firm. Steve's mother was pleased to baby-sit her first grandchild.

Jennifer's parents suspected that something was wrong when Jennifer was an infant. Their concerns were brought to the attention of their physician when Jennifer was six months old. The pediatrician told them not to worry that their daughter was alert and bright and was one of those calm infants who did not startle easily. This diagnosis was a relief to Paula and Steve who had been afraid that their daughter was deaf. Steve's mother urged the young couple to seek a second opinion because her daily contact with Jennifer convinced her that something was wrong. Paula agreed but decided to postpone further evaluation.

The parents' nagging worries continued as Jennifer matured physically, yet failed to develop speech and language. When Jennifer was two years old and with Paula and Steve's permission, Grandmother took Jennifer to an early childhood evaluation screening where she was urged to set up an appointment with an otolaryngologist. Paula took her daughter to the doctor and was not surprised that an audiological evaluation was requested. Jennifer was difficult for the audiologist to test because she would not sit still and cooperate. A repeat-test two weeks later was also inconclusive and an ABR test was recommended. Steve and Paula accompanied Jennifer to the large medical center where the test was conducted and where their worst fears were confirmed. The nagging suspicions ended and the reality of the situation was exposed. Jennifer had a severe to profound bilateral hearing loss of unknown etiology that could be treated with the use of aids. The parents were unable to recall if any other information was given to them on the day of the diagnosis.

At this time, Paula was four months pregnant. Feeling overwhelmed by all that had to be done for Jennifer, and with Steve's agreement and support, she quit her job thus creating a significant loss in income for the family as well as removing her from her support system of friends. Steve's mother agreed to help whenever needed. Paula's mother and stepfather remained somewhat distant from the crisis apparently afraid that their expressions of worry would make matters worse.

Jennifer was fitted with aids which she wore inconsistently. The power struggle that accompanied the insertion of the aids was an ordeal for parent and child. The audiologist suggested aural habilitation and a referral was made to a speech-language pathologist.

When Paula called for an appointment, she was told that an alternative service delivery model was available that included the entire family in the treatment process. This idea appealed to Paula and the decision was made to convene Paula, Steve, Grandma, and Jennifer since these were the family members who had the most contact with Jennifer. An evening appointment was arranged to accommodate Steve's work schedule.

The initial session revealed the parents' extreme frustration with their inability to communicate effectively with their daughter. They also expressed concern about difficulty disciplining a child who did not respond to speech and language and worried about Jennifer's future interaction with other children. They had been advised by a family friend, who had once known a deaf person, "not let her use that funny sign language." Their confusion had been compounded by conflicting advice. Their family physician told them to avoid hearing aids because Jennifer's hearing could be further damaged. The advice of the audiologist and otolaryngologist was to use aids along with auditory training. Paula cried as she expressed her frustration about this confusion. Steve comforted her as the clinician listened calmly and empathically to her concerns. Jennifer ran around the room eliciting frequent and always unsuccessful attempts by Steve and Grandma to calm her down.

In spite of the chaos and grief that pervaded the first session, a goal was established that seemed to make sense to everyone present. Jennifer would be helped to recognize and use words that had everyday usefulness to her as she interacted with her parents and grandmother. This goal was isomorphic to the family's desire to develop communication with their daughter.

An assignment was designed to fit this goal using the resources displayed by the family during the initial part of the interview. Grandmother, mother, and father were all asked to pay special attention to those times when a specific word or phrase would aid communication and to make a list of all of those words and phrases. When the assignment was suggested, the parents immediately began to discuss words and phrases that could appear on the list. They were heartened by the suggestion that effective communication might be possible. The parents were also asked to have a serious discussion about their desires for alternate communication options so that these could be incorporated into treatment. The clinician stressed that it was critical that they be comfortable with whichever option they chose. They were also told that any communication decision could be modified to fit the family's and Jennifer's unique needs as treatment progressed. The clinician described a total communication approach that she thought was best for Jennifer given her severe to profound hearing loss.

Formal language testing was not done because the clinician was unable to create a shared focus of attention. The clinician, however, observed several spontaneous interactions showing Jennifer's out-of-bounds behavior and her parents' and grandmother's unsuccessful attempts to control her. It seemed very clear that Jennifer was not attending to or understanding her family's disciplinary directives!

Steve, Paula, Grandma, Jennifer, *and* Grandpa arrived for the next session bearing a long list of words and phrases that they had developed. In addition, the family members identified gestures that Jennifer was using that conveyed meaning. Steve and Paula expressed relief that something was getting started and said that they wanted to try total communication with Jennifer. They also remarked that they seemed to be communicating better with Jennifer already because she was "paying more attention to us." Since the clinician was familiar with Signed English, she asked the parents permission to use this sign method along with other aural rehabilitation techniques. The parents readily agreed. During the week they had also decided to attempt to make better use of the hearing aids and had made some headway in getting Jennifer to wear them for successively longer periods of time.

As treatment progressed, Jennifer's language skills improved dramatically and a concomitant change in her behavior was noted. The parents reported that her speech was unintelligible to people outside the family, but they were thrilled that they were able to understand several of the words and phrases that she was using. She learned to wear the aids without complaint, perhaps signifying her parents' acceptance of their use. Both parents expressed concern about the way strangers seemed to stare at Jennifer when the family was out in public and stated that they were reluctant to communicate with Signed

English in the presence of strangers.

Steve and Grandma continued to meet with the clinician following the birth of Jennifer's brother Timmy who began attending sessions with his family when he was two months old. After ten months of treatment, the family, with the help of the clinician, had learned developmentally appropriate communication techniques and were in the focusing outward stage of the grieving process.

Unfortunately, a different problem emerged creating new family stress. Steve and Paula's desire to have their three-year-old daughter enrolled in preschool so that she could interact more with other children presented a different family dilemma. The local special education district wanted Jennifer enrolled in a preschool located an hour's bus ride away from the family home. Steve and Paula felt that Jennifer was too young for such a trip and wanted her enrolled in a preschool for hearing children closer to home. Although unsupported by the special education personnel who had been advising them, the family went ahead and enrolled Jennifer in the preschool of their choice.

The clinician worked with the family to obtain an auditory trainer and explained its use to the preschool teacher who was eager to help. The family was unsuccessful in obtaining financial support for hearing-impaired itinerant services and Jennifer was isolated from most of her peers. The preschool teacher, however, decided to introduce her entire class of children to some basic signs and consulted with the parents and the clinician as she developed and learned how to use these signs. In addition, the clinician worked with the teacher to help her make full use of Jennifer's aided auditory ability. Other professionals offered several new pieces of advice at this time ranging from, "She should be enrolled in a school for the deaf so she can become part of the deaf community," to "You shouldn't be teaching her sign language, she'll never be able to relate to hearing people if she doesn't learn to talk." This kind of advice, along with the family's introduction to the overwhelming array of educational decisions that they now knew they would have to make, elicited feelings of confusion, anger, and disappointment that were freely expressed by both Steve and Paula. They had thought that, "the worst was over" but, instead, were beginning their long voyage into the social service network maze and were, once again, overwhelmed by the decision-making responsibilities that confronted them.

As the family worked with the clinician to develop Jennifer's communicative abilities, the maternal grandparents were also enlisted to participate in treatment from time to time. Jennifer's intelligibility continued to improve as the family learned to reinforce her speech and as they struggled to develop their Signed English skills by attending sign language classes. Although change was gradual, viewing of videotapes from former sessions encouraged the family as they became aware of the ability of their family to effectively communicate with Jennifer.

Speech-language treatment continued although the sessions were less frequent since all family members were able to reinforce and assist Jennifer during normal daily activities. Jennifer was functioning adequately in the mainstream preschool, but Steve and Paula remained concerned that this might not be the best placement for her. Paula wanted to return to work but delayed that move until critical decisions about Jennifer's school placement were made. In spite of the continuing stress associated with Jennifer's hearing impairment, the parent's were empowered to fully parent their daughter. They took great delight in this and also enjoyed the pleasures to be found watching the growth and development of two active preschool children.

SUMMARY

Families with young children must accommodate to the rapidly changing physical, social, and emotional needs of their children. The well-being of the child is powerfully influenced by the well-being of his/her parents. Therefore adults must assure that their own needs are met. When a child is born with special needs these developmental tasks are complicated by the extra attention that the child must receive and the decisions that must be made relative to professional intervention.

Involving the family in treatment ensures their rightful place in the decision-making process and enhances the clinician's opportunities to create assignments that will benefit the child. The Family Based Treatment model can be used to involve family members in the treatment of a variety of communicative disorders.

CHAPTER 11

APPLICATION TO FAMILIES WITH MIDDLE CHILDHOOD AND ADOLESCENT CHILDREN

When children enter school, roles and responsibilities within the family shift and the family moves into a new phase of the childhood stage. Families with several children begin this change with the oldest child's advancement to school and enter a new phase when the child enters adolescence. Adolescence, the fourth family development stage (Carter & McGoldrick, 1989), continues until the family begins launching the oldest child. The developmental model delineates the beginning of a transition based on the age of the oldest child, but in many families subsequent children necessitate that attention be paid to younger children that are following the same developmental path.

FAMILY DEVELOPMENTAL FACTORS

The elementary school years tend to be less stressful for parents than the pre-school years as children become increasingly independent, more facile in tending to their physical needs, and competent in peer relationships. In addition, the transition to school separates family members for increasingly longer periods of time during which the child develops personal competence. This relieves the parents from some of the intensity of their earlier caregiving duties.

When adolescence begins, many families become destabilized as new values, emotions, expectations, and personal styles are introduced into the family by the child and his/her peers. It may be impossible to "raise" teenagers. Perhaps, instead, they raise parents, and in the end the parents are wiser and more competent people as a result of all they have learned from their children. This chapter will focus on the early and later school years including the adolescent transition. The case examples will describe family treatment with children having language, articulation, and phonological problems.

Parent-Child Interaction

Child-rearing is a process that requires the setting of appropriate boundaries while also encouraging the child's independence and personal decision-making within those boundaries. Infants are closely monitored, and the boundaries are tightly drawn around the mother, child, and other significant family members. The protection shown in these early years is necessary and appropriate. In well-functioning families as the child matures, boundaries are gradually expanded until the individual reaches young adulthood and imposed family boundaries are no longer necessary since the individual is now able to make his/her own personal life decisions. The school years are critical to the child as personal competence, peer relationships, sibling relationships, and an identity that is separate from the family's is developed. Competent parents understand this and keep an appropriate balance between the imposition of boundaries and personal decision-making freedom. As the child matures, mistakes are made, lessons are learned, and successes are experienced. This gradual unfolding of life experiences interfaces with the child's developmental abilities and a mature, responsible adult eventually emerges often surprising his/her beleaguered parents.

Negotiating boundaries and personal freedom may be especially difficult for parents and children when special needs must be considered. The natural protectiveness of a mother for a preschool daughter who is deaf may persist into the school-age years as the difficult decisions about safe boundaries and personal freedom are established, changed, and re-established. Decisions relative to the restrictions placed on a ten-year-old with cerebral palsy must be made without impeding growth and maturation. The issues of adolescent sexuality, often problematic for parents whose children are "normal," must be confronted and explored as the child with special needs matures. The development of a personal identity, critical to every maturing individual, will not occur without trial and error, conflict, and parental sorrow as parents are once again reminded that their child's progress does not fall nicely into the "normal" developmental norms. As each developmental milestone is approached, the parents must readjust their expectations to fit the capabilities of their child. This can be a complicated, difficult, and rewarding task.

Sibling Interaction

Sibling relationships take on new significance at this time. If the parents were sometimes overwhelmed by the needs of their child with a communicative disorder during the early years, they may now experience a sense of relief as he/she is enrolled in school and more free time is available to the adults in the family. This change may awaken the realization that other children in the family had not received the attention they were due during the stressful early years. Siblings, sensing their parents' renewed energy, may express resentment about the attention paid to brother or sister. This occurs now since mother and father are strong enough to handle such information. An older sibling who takes on the role of the responsible child, may inadvertently become a third "parent" creating expectations well beyond reason when considered from the perspective of the older sibling's own developmental needs. Siblings often share the work associated with the added pressures of communicative delay and disability and, generally, benefit from the attitudes and abilities derived from these experiences. However, care must be taken to keep an appropriate balance between the older sibling's involvement with a brother or sister who is communicatively disabled or delayed and his/her own normal developmental tasks. Family Based Treatment offers an excellent opportunity to assist in this process while also benefiting the child with special needs.

We always invite the siblings of our speech-language clients to attend the family sessions. Younger siblings tend to attend every session while older siblings attend when the meetings do not conflict with their normal adolescent activities. The siblings are wonderful resources as we plan and develop treatment procedures. Their presence makes it possible to monitor sibling involvement so that it is balanced with developmental needs and parents' expectations and desires. Sister or brother's fresh and unaffected desire to offer suggestions adds interest and fun to the family meetings. When sibling rivalry erupts, we can assess it's impact on the communicative disorder, ask parents how they like to handle these conflicts, and normalize the disagreements so that siblings are encouraged to develop their own problem solving style within appropriate parentally established boundaries. Our experience clearly shows that school-age siblings appreciate being included in the treatment process. They gain, sometimes for the first time, an understanding of the communicative disorder and are appreciated members of the habilitative team.

Peer Interaction

The importance of peer relationships is magnified for families having a child with disabilities. The strong desire of all people at every age level to develop meaningful friendships is particularly imposing during later childhood and early adolescence. The child who is developmentally disabled and who wants to have friends and relate well to peers may be rebuffed and forced to deal with the pain of rejection. Although not all children and adolescents with special needs are confronted with this problem, it is more common than for children who are developing normally. A mother of one of our adolescent clients tried, without success, to arrange a prom date for her daughter. She wanted her daughter to attend the prom with a boy having similar special needs. Her sensitive attention to this task failed, and the disappointment everyone experienced rippled through the speech-language treatment process.

Extended Family Interaction

Extended family members continue to be important to the client and his/her parents during the school years. Grandparents start to notice their own age-related changes and adult children begin to shift their focus to the needs of their parents. This happens while parents are simultaneously dealing with the behaviors of unpredictable adolescents. The fortunate families who have assessed and dealt with their differences related to the raising of the child with special needs will enjoy the support and continued help offered by grandparents, aunts, uncles, and other extended family members on whom the family has come to rely. Those who have not openly acknowledged and confronted these differences may experience an increasing tension relative to unsolicited advice and criticism from these and other relatives during the school-age years. In most cases, however, the speech-language clinician will find cooperative relationships between generations. The consultative expertise of the third generation is welcomed by most family members and the clinician as well.

We are often surprised and always delighted to meet third and fourth generation family members that our families bring to family treatment sessions and are careful to include them in the process of the session. In these cases, we believe that the parents are aware of the importance of everyone understanding the efforts being made to create speech-language change and want to share this with their child's grandparents. Involving three generations in treatment is not limited to a particular economic or social class. Most families seem to appreciate the support that can be offered by grandparents. In other cases, the conflict between generations becomes evident as treatment proceeds and this is always a clue for us to ask the parents if they think it would be helpful to invite the grandparents to a meeting. When agreement to do this is reached, we are careful to structure the session so that the parents are supported in their parental role. This includes asking the parents to provide an explanation of the treatment that has been developed and positively commenting on the parents' participation. Every time that we have arranged a session of this sort, the tension appears to be decreased between generations relative to the communicative disorder. The grandparents love for their grandchild is accessed, and they are able to experience first hand the parental competence of their adult children as treatment procedures are described.

Siblings, extended family members, and even parents are not included in all sessions as the client matures into adolescence. Adolescent independence is reinforced when individual sessions are held with the permission of the parents and at the desire of the adolescent. Attempts to wrench the child away from an "overinvolved" family into independence are replaced with cooperative planning and mutual appreciation for the adolescent's maturational process. This mutual planning often leads the family to request that the adolescent be allowed to work on the problem independently. The adolescent usually prefers such an arrangement and individual sessions are integrated into the Family Based Treatment process.

CASE STUDIES

Articulation/Phonological Disorders

Errors in phoneme production are among those communicative problems that require the most structured and systematic approach to treatment. Treatment is characterized by small, orderly steps and consistent, discriminating use of reinforcement in order to shape the desired behavior. The effectiveness of interventions is obvious to the careful listener and the behavior of the client clearly guides the clinician in the development of successive interventions. As we apply the Family Based Treatment model to families having a member with one of these disorders, we are struck with how often the extent of generalization surpasses our expectations and with family members' ability to incorporate effective interventions into everyday activities. The latter is especially interesting since we traditionally view our procedures as requiring near-laboratory conditions in terms of the precision with which they should be introduced. Further, we do not usually think of phonology in terms of interactions as we do language and stuttering. This increases the challenge.

A very important principle that emerged was to assign activities which the child would clearly be able to do. This means eliciting and practicing phonemes in contexts in which there is absolute certainty that the child and family will be successful. Family members are not asked to shape behavior as a speech-language pathologist would do or to make subtle or difficult distinctions between different productions of the same sound. Assignments are carefully developed to be isomorphic to each family's activities and resources. Clearly, if family members are to reinforce appropriate behavior, the behavior must be easily discernible in the course of natural interactions in noisy, and sometimes even chaotic, environments. Family members should be rewarded for their work just as the child is rewarded for new appropriate behavior. Assignments are idiosyncratic to each family and each child and are based upon rewarding success for behavior that is near maximum in terms of effort possible in a natural setting. Further, goals must be clearly understood by family members, and the first goal is nearly always one which may be reached in several sessions. This is an important factor in empowering families and demonstrating that they can be successful. This same notion is a traditional principle that clinicians have applied to individual clients for many years. We merely adapt it to families. Within the context of the agreed-upon and achievable goal, each session consists of reviewing progress and searching for the maximum successful behavior possible. Still, the behavior has to be easily detectable to the family so that it can be rewarded appropriately.

Sometimes the child's immediate environment is other than the natural family. In this case the system is defined to include the significant people who interact with the client on a daily basis. Tom was a child like this. He had been removed from the home of his natural family and placed in a residential setting for boys whose families were not able to manage or care for them. The staff at the home was concerned about Tom's speech and made an appointment for an evaluation. Because Tom's records showed that he had been seen by the authors when he was younger, we were asked to re-evaluate him. Actually, we had seen him only one time when he was much younger. His family had been referred to us and we met for one session but they were unable to continue as is often the case when parents are distressed and must struggle to meet their most basic needs. When we saw Tom six years later, he was a sullen, frightened, taciturn thirteen-year-old whose speech was unintelligible. He was accompanied by a representative of the home who obviously was concerned about him and attempted to interact with him. Tom did not reciprocate.

During this first session we listened to Tom's speech, but the majority of the time was spent attempting to define an appropriate interactive system with which to work. We were told that Tom's natural family was not available and could not be a part of that system. The representative who accompanied Tom neither knew him nor would be one who would interact with him other than to bring him to sessions. Because the residential setting was in a city some distance from the clinic in which we were working, the representative indicated that Tom would be limited to one session per week. At the same time, however, the staff who interacted with Tom wanted him to receive services. The representative thought that one counselor in particular interacted well with Tom and Tom with him. We ended the session with the understanding that the representative would speak with that counselor and attempt to arrange for him to accompany Tom to the next and subsequent weekly sessions.

Tom arrived the next week and was accompanied by a young man who identified himself as one of Tom's counselors. While Tom was far from effusive, there was an obvious difference in his manner especially in response to the counselor. The counselor described Tom as being much like he was when he was young, and he believed that if Tom could develop a better self image, a natural result would be improved interactions with others. The counselor also described how Tom was teased and intimidated by two of the other boys. Tom agreed and named the boys. The counselor also discussed things he did in an attempt to help Tom. These included asking Tom to practice words that were especially difficult for him to say, having Tom practice saying the names of other counselors, and asking Tom to repeat the words "can of pop" when Tom requested this. Tom indicated that he was willing to do this and even liked practicing with the counselor. These activities were clear resources which could be elaborated upon and refined. An additional resource emerged with the counselor's description of his efforts to enhance Tom's place in the hierarchy of peers at the home. We agreed that the counselor would accompany Tom to sessions and that they would work together in the residential setting. We also agreed that he would garner the support of other counselors and even some of the boys who interacted with Tom. With this, the system was defined as Tom, the counselor, and the clinician. Subsystems, with which we would not come in contact, would include the counselor, Tom, and other counselors; the counselor, Tom, and other boys at the home; and various combinations of members of these groups.

Tom's speech was characterized by poor use of rhythm and intonation, deletion of final sounds, consistent use of a glottal stop for /g/ in prevocalic and intervocalic positions, omission of liquids or substitution of a plosive for a liquid, and many other inconsistent errors. Tom was stimulable for most sounds in isolation and in consonant-vowel syllables.

The counselor was a participant in the evaluation. The clinician administered the articulation test, did stimulability testing, and elicited other speech samples, but he also engaged the counselor in attempting to elicit correct sounds, syllables, and words. The counselor was obviously comfortable in the situation and rewarded Tom well. He also found the idea of thinking about how sounds are produced fascinating and interesting. The counselor's genuine interest seemed to elicit interest from Tom. We viewed this as another resource. As we discussed goals, the counselor turned to Tom from time to time and asked him to repeat particular phrases, words, and sounds. Tom's counselor had noticed that the rhythm of Tom's speech was poor. The many articulation errors, including use of glottal stops, contributed to this. The counselor requested that whatever we did, it should be something with which Tom would be successful so that Tom's self-esteem might be improved.

We decided to delay setting a goal relative to a particular phoneme or phoneme group and, rather, have a general initial goal of improving the rhythm of Tom's speech and his awareness of the rhythm of speech. We found four, two and three word phrases which Tom could say perfectly. The assignment was for the counselor to elicit these from Tom in many different situations making it as spontaneous and as much fun as possible, and to reward Tom appropriately. Tom agreed to participate in this activity and to cooperate fully. He was obviously pleased with how he sounded when he said these phrases and with his counselor's praise and pleasure when he did so. A second assignment was for the counselor to pay attention to other phrases that sounded perfect when Tom said them and to bring a list of these to the next session.

It should be noted that both assignments focused on positive features of Tom's ability. Since, as Wilcox (1989) points out, remediation inherently calls attention to deficits as the focus or topic of emphasis, it is important to assign interventions that capitalize on clients' abilities and strengths and to gradually nudge performance forward. Families and clients who experience success and appropriate reward become empowered to undertake more and greater challenges. At the same time, they are less likely to be overcome by discouragement when an intervention is not successful.

Tom, his counselor, and a peer of Tom's from the home accompanied Tom to the third session. Both Tom and his counselor had enjoyed interjecting the phrases into natural practice situations, and the counselor had interested some of the other boys in aspects of speech production. This allied them with Tom in a new way. Not only were Tom's peers discouraged from teasing him but Tom even gained new friends and supporters who appreciated Tom's new ability to "talk normally." The counselor had heard several additional phrases which Tom said well. We refined these during the session, had the counselor ask Tom to say them, and with Tom's permission, also engaged Tom's friend in this activity. All showed pleasure with Tom's "normal speech," and the assignment was continued for one more week.

At the fourth session, Tom noticed that what he did to sound normal was to exaggerate the movements of his mouth. We talked at some length about exactly what he felt he had been doing when his speech sounded good. Tom and the counselor had collaborated in developing a list of additional phrases which Tom could say perfectly. These were added to the list for Tom to practice using the techniques he now understood and was able to use intentionally. We also elicited a /g/ from Tom which had been difficult previously even though he was able to produce /k/. Tom and his counselor practiced Tom's production of /g/ and it was evident that even if Tom "lost" it, he and the counselor would be able to use the /k/ sound as a guide to "find" it again. A second assignment, in addition to practicing the phrases, was for Tom to practice producing /g/ (combined with a schwa) with his counselor. Reinforcing came so naturally for the counselor that he hardly had to be reminded that this was a very important part of the practice. A goal was set for Tom to be able to produce /g/ at will.

By the sixth session Tom was able to use the /g/ correctly in six words. He and his counselor had practiced increasing the speed with which he said these words and used the technique of combining them into artificial phrases with different rhythmical sequences. This was a method of combining the two assignments and using one to aid the other in a novel way. Both Tom and his counselor were rewarded for this innovation.

By this time Tom's speech intelligibility had improved. His interpersonal relations were markedly better. For the first time, he participated in events and initiated interaction with peers. He also walked and sat more deliberately, held his head so that he could look forward rather than down, and appropriately varied the expression on his face. Tom, his counselor, other staff at the home, and even many peers were pleased with these changes. Tom was reaping the rewards of his new interpersonal skills through intentional responses of others, but also in their unplanned, spontaneous reactions.

Treatment with Tom was terminated shortly thereafter when he moved out of the state. The interactive system that had become the unit of treatment was clearly different from the traditional family.

Members of Tom's system responded creatively and resourcefully to our attempts to use their many resources. Assignments were isomorphic to the lifestyle of the residents and were created in a polyocular manner. This gave Tom's counselor a new and interesting way of thinking about speech. In all, we had seven sessions over a period of two months. Unfortunately, the details of Tom's move were not available to us, so we were not able to link with others who might be serving him in his new home. Tom's speech changed less than his pragmatics of interaction, but we all found great satisfaction with the results of our systemic treatment process.

When the problem is simply articulatory in nature, it might seem that family participation would be unnecessary. Yet in our experience, that is not necessarily the case. April, for example, was twelve years old and had a persistent lateral distortion of the "sh" sound. She had received speech-language services on an individual basis for five years. While other articulation errors were corrected during that time, the "sh" distortion persisted. In fact, the "sh" distortion had shown little change even after over one year of individual services focused on that sound alone. April's articulation was normal in all other respects.

April and her family were referred in hopes that family participation would make a difference. Since the problem was well defined and limited in scope we agreed to having one parent involved in each session. We did, however, want both parents involved rather than have the same parent attend each session. April's mother participated in the first and subsequent sessions and, fortunately, after six sessions (and before the father was able to attend a session) April was using the "sh" sound accurately in conversational speech and was dismissed.

As with Tom, we wanted to build upon success and give assignments that could be carried out easily in the context of the family environment. At the first session the clinician was able to elicit a correct production of the "sh" sound in isolation, but April was not able to produce this with ease. It was clear that it was too early to assign April's mother to elicit the sound from April or for April to practice the sound. For this reason, the assignment given to the family at the first session was to let April *hear* the "sh" sound a lot but not to ask her to say it. Family members were to make the sound in isolation many times during the day in a playful way as they saw April and interacted with her. They were also to exaggerate the sound in words that came up in conversation with April and to intentionally say words containing the sound as they interacted with April. All of this was to be done in an enjoyable and friendly manner. No attempts were to be made to have April imitate family members' productions and she was not to be asked to produce the sound or say words containing the sound.

When April and her mother arrived for the second session, they described how the assignment had been implemented. Both April and her mother agreed that no one had asked her to say anything. April, however, admitted that she had privately practiced the sound and that hearing it so much may have helped her. Clearly, something had helped her because she was able to find and produce the sound accurately and with ease. Her mother was surprised and pleased, and April received genuine acclaim from her.

From this point through the next four sessions, April was asked to let her family hear many productions of the sound (first in isolation and increasingly in syllables and words), and to practice increasing the speed with which she was able to read a list of words each containing an "sh" sound. In all cases, the interventions and practice were to be enjoyable and carried out during normal family activities, not during special times set aside for practice.

At the sixth session, April's mother and April

both reported that the correct sound was part of April's natural articulatory repertoire. Both felt that no more sessions were necessary; the clinician agreed. One year later, April had maintained accurate use of the sound and had normal speech.

We are sure that the years of individual treatment that preceded our work with April laid the groundwork for rapid change. However, the involvement of family members (her mother and other family members recruited by her mother) completed the project. This change in the treatment model; the incorporation of interventions, practice, and reinforcement into everyday natural interactions; and the participation of the family in treatment seemed to be the factors that led to April's rapid success.

Language Disorders

Language is a complex issue and although we advocate that families participate in the treatment of all types of language problems, it is understood that some aspects of language disorders will test the creative strategizing abilities of clinicians more than others. We have been very successful in helping a family effect change in its child's use of plurals, for example. Improving the same child's use of verb tense, however, was more difficult and frustrating. Plurals, as the child's parents pointed out, are easy; verb tense is complicated. Family interventions with plurals were easily made into enjoyable activities that could be carried out during and after meals, while watching television, and during the usual interactions of everyday life at home. All adults and older children in the family could easily make contributions because all understood the concept and could describe it. Interventions to improve verb tense was more challenging because many more grammatical rules are involved and more variations present themselves.

Ken's family helped him perfect his use of plurals. For example, dad made up games such as having Ken guess how many pennies dad had in his hand: "How many pennies do I have?" asked dad. "I think you have one penny in your hand." "No, I have more than one penny. How many pennies do you think I have?" "I think you have four pennies." "No, I have more than that, I have eight pennies. How many pennies did I have?" "You had eight pennies." "Good job, Ken!"

Ken's older brother also made up a game. He combined a number with an object to which Ken responded by changing plural to singular or singular to plural. For example, when Ken's brother said, "two ducks," Ken would respond, "one duck." This game was incorporated into mealtimes, when encountering one another in the house, in the car, etc. Both Ken and his brother enjoyed the game; Ken's brother especially liked to catch Ken "off guard" and surprise him with an intervention. Obviously, this was a playful family; different activities could be developed for families who spent more time reading books, engaging in physical activities, visiting grandparents, etc.

In our culture, the first natural response to a communicative disorder may be to ask the person questions! This seems to occur as a natural reaction independent of the problem or age of the person with the communicative difficulty. The second-most common response to children with language disorders may be to correct their speech. Since this is antithetical to building upon success and to reinforcing that success, it is important to creatively strategize with families in a manner that results in proactive, positive-outcome interventions built into family lifestyles.

Susan, for example, was a first grader whose correct use of past tense regular and irregular verbs was inconsistent. She lived with her mother, her mother's parents, and a nine year old sister. That group, along with the clinician, made up the interactive system. Everyone attended nearly all of the sessions, so access to the system was good.

All three adults had a tendency to ask Susan questions, to tell her what to say, and to correct grammatical errors they heard in Susan's spontaneous speech. Susan reacted to these attempts to help her by becoming sullen, by shouting (eg., "don't tell me" or "no"), by withdrawing from the situation (eg., crawling under the table, leaving the room, going to another part of the room and covering her ears with her hands), and/or by physically striking the "guilty" family member. These interactions seemed to be perpetuating the problem.

Family resources included a strong desire to help Susan improve her use of language, helpful grandparents who added to the number of adults who loved and cared for Susan, a strong positive relationship between Susan and her grandmother who enjoyed doing household chores together, and family members who enjoyed looking at books and reading with Susan. We focused our attention on these resources, incorporated them into our creative strategizing, and highlighted them in discussions with the family. Initially, we ignored those interactions that seemed to be perpetuating the problem, but when they did not change, we discussed them with the family. The use of counseling techniques was an important component of these discussions.

Assignments consisted of activities which built on family resources. We stressed that Susan should hear a lot of past tense verbs and be put in situations in which family members would use them for her to hear. Examples included emphasizing and even repeating short sentences and phrases with past tense verbs when looking at books; having grandmother review the house work she and Susan had done together emphasizing each past tense verb and repeating the phrase once or twice; and having Susan and her older sister review their day with one of the adults. When the use of questions, corrections, and requests to imitate did not subside, we gave an assignment to pay attention to the number of questions and corrections the adults used with Susan and to notice Susan's reaction to these. This was not intended to let the adults see how "bad" they were. Rather, the intent was to lay the groundwork for the adults to notice Susan's responses to other types of interventions and for an assignment to use techniques other than questioning and correcting. The earlier assignments, to let Susan hear her family members use and emphasize past tense verbs, was in preparation for asking them not to correct, ask questions, or request imitations. When family members are given assignments that include active interventions involving new ways of interacting, it may be easier for them to stop or reduce the interactions that perpetuate the problem because they are doing something new rather than merely trying not to do something.

After several sessions, family members began suggesting other activities which involved the use of past tense verbs. They had, for example, looked at family photographs with Susan. She enjoyed this, and since the photos involved past activities, past tense verbs flowed easily and naturally. The grandparents had developed a game in which one of them did an action. Then, together with Susan, the other grandparent described the action (eg., you closed the door, you pushed your chair, etc.). At that point, we believed that we could assign them to repeat correctly phrases with past tense verbs that they heard Susan use incorrectly. They were not to call these to her attention, but merely to restate them correctly once or twice. Also, they were asked to reinforce those which they heard Susan use correctly. Another activity involved the adults audiotaping stories to which Susan listened, became familiar, and then retold. Still another activity was to read books that were familiar to Susan and to pause before saying some of the past tense verbs to let

Susan say them and be rewarded for her successful use of the past tense.

Susan and her family enjoyed carrying out the assignments that we developed together. Interactions with Susan no longer consisted primarily of questions, corrections, and requests to imitate. In fact, these were rarely heard after five or six sessions. Susan's behavior improved along with the elimination of the interactions that she had come to dislike. Most importantly, Susan's use of past tense verbs improved and correct usage became incorporated into her spontaneous speech.

SUMMARY

During the school years children gradually become less dependent on their parents. Sibling and peer relationships increase in importance, and as the child enters adolescence, issues associated with sexuality and impending adult independence begin to emerge. Families must learn how to allow the child to expand his/her boundaries while also maintaining appropriate personal control. Parental decision-making relative to the child with special needs continues as families learn to relate to schools and to the larger social service system.

Family Based Treatment encourages developmentally appropriate sibling participation, parental and grandparental involvement, peer interaction, and the developing independence of the child or adolescent. When the child or adolescent is not living with immediate family members, other significant people from the child's environment may be successfully included in the treatment process.

CHAPTER 12

APPLICATION TO ADULTS AND THEIR FAMILIES

The launching process begins when children reach age eighteen, finish high school, and move into the world of work and/or post secondary education. The between families stage (Carter and McGoldrick, 1980) now commences for young adult children, and a new generation of adults evolves. These changes are accompanied by the development of adult intimate relationships, as well as decisions relating to sexuality, marriage, and childbearing. While these developmentally critical young adult changes are taking place, parents move on to relationship and career experiences infused with a fresh sense of freedom.

FAMILY DEVELOPMENTAL FACTORS OF ADULTHOOD

Couples who are in their first marriage identify the launching stage as the most maritally satisfying of all the family developmental stages (Anderson, Russell & Schumm, 1983; Glenn, 1975; Rollins & Feldman, 1970). Single parents gradually experience a lessening of financial and caregiving responsibility and may, for the first time in many years, have time to attend fully to their own adult needs. The launching stage is filled with numerous family exits and entrances as people leave, return, and leave again often accompanied by friends, fiances, marital partners, and grandchildren. The parental expectation that the launching process will be smooth and brief is usually unfulfilled, particularly when children participate in post- secondary education or protracted career exploration requiring financial support well beyond age twenty-one, the usual age of independence. Families with several children may be launching one or more children while also dealing with school-aged and adolescent offspring. Launching interfaces with the later years stage as grandparents and great-grandparents begin to require additional attention and support. The complexities and challenges of family life continue often accompanied by unanticipated events that demand the reassertion of problem solving skills.

When all children are launched, parents enter their child-free years and begin planning for retirement. As parents (grandparents) approach age 65, the family begins its last stage, the later years. Advancements in medical care allow people to live longer, the quality of life has improved for most older families, and many people remain active well into their eighth and ninth decades (Vander Zanden, 1989). Furthermore, variations in temperament, cognitive ability, physical stamina, and social interests between people of similar ages create a mosaic of behavior that is decidedly heterogeneous. For example, two normal seventy-five-year-olds will vary in motor, cognitive, and social ability to a much greater extent than will two adolescents. Our seventeen-year-old son noted this variation as he admired the strength and stamina of a seventy-seven year old man who was part of a 400 mile, weeklong bicycle tour across the State of Iowa. Our son was impressed by the gentleman's physical ability as well as by his "old-fashioned" single speed bicycle, quite unlike the high tech vehicles ridden by many of the adolescent, young adult, and middle-aged adult participants. Almost any healthy seventeen-year-old could manage such a tour; fewer seventy-seven-year-olds could survive this arduous journey. Sensitivity to this tremendous variation in individual ability and circumstance must be integrated into the speech-language pathologist's clinical skills repertoire when working with older adults.

Family life during the launching and moving on stage, as well as during the later years, is characterized by many

Application to Adults and Their Families

interwoven events. The spiraling generations weave a tapestry of complex relationships that change with each new generation yet show intricately-related patterns that are intergenerationally connected as grandchildren and great-grandchildren are born and new generations are formed. The "last" stage is final for one part of the generational spiral but not for the family system since every stage of the life cycle is interrelated to every other stage. The interconnectedness of the family is powerfully experienced during these "last" two stages of the family life cycle. This chapter will review the impact of disability on these stages and describe family involvement in the treatment of communicative disorders associated with aphasia and mental retardation.

Shifting Parent-Young Adult Interaction

Independence stands out as a major goal to be achieved during the launching stage of the family life cycle. This goal includes the physical independence experienced when a child establishes an apartment, moves to a college dormitory, or continues to live at home (with fewer restrictions than were imposed previously) while preparing for financial independence. Sooner or later, personal mastery of career skills appropriate to the early adult years occurs and financial credibility is established thus freeing parents of the financial burdens of the early launching stage. Intimate relationships are explored and developed and the young adult begins to make decisions that may or may not correspond to the decisions made by the parental generation during its early adult years.

Concurrently, parents become independent of childrearing responsibilities and new opportunities for their own personal and relationship change and growth are created. A mutual separation between parents and young adult children occurs and is experienced as exciting, challenging, and perhaps foreboding as the young person succeeds, flounders, reorganizes, and moves on, eventually establishing complete physical, career, and financial independence. In some families, parents are confronted with a returning launched adult who is going through a divorce, has lost his or her job, or requires special care related to an unexpected problem such as alcoholism. Unanticipated developmental disruptions increase family stress and create dilemmas that once again demand the use of problem solving skills.

Developmental disability has a powerful impact on emerging independence. Some families in which a young adult has a developmental disability will traverse the launching transition with the same equanimity found in most other families and will, after four or five years, be pleased and sometimes surprised to discover that their child has moved successfully into adult independence. This independence may take a different form from that of a nondisabled person but it is achieved. Other families may not be able to achieve independence for themselves and their adult child for financial reasons or because of the severity of the disability.

Two family issues may be particularly evident to the speech-language pathologist during this transition. First, an accident or illness may create a permanent disability and serious, unexpected individual and family developmental disruption. Second, family disruption may appear to be evident in the parent-child relationship of the developmentally disabled young adult who has been disabled since childhood as adult independence becomes an issue. Both of these may seem to create transitional upheaval. Grieving and loss are powerfully related to these issues. Let us now turn our attention to the developmental concerns related to each of these issues.

Unexpected Illness or Accident

The sudden disruption of an accident or illness pulls the family back into the life of the young adult just as he or she has begun or just completed the transition to adulthood. Head injury, for example, can occur at any time in the life cycle, but the incidence is highest for males between fifteen and thirty-five and peaks in the fifteen to twenty-four year old range (Rollin, 1987). The family's energy is immediately focused on the preservation of life. The brief sense of elation that is experienced when life is assured is followed by days, months, years, and sometimes a lifetime of concern for the quality of life that their loved one might achieve (DePompei, 1987). Furthermore, variations in complications, ranging from minor to major, make each case unique and require clinician sensitivity to the idiosyncratic responses of the client and his/her family members as effects are assessed and treated.

Attention to intergenerational issues is imperative. In the case of a head-injured person who is married with young children, the young family is irrevocably changed as spouse and children attempt to accommodate to their "new" family member. If the young adult is not married or if divorce occurs following the injury, aging parents are powerfully impacted by the expectation that they abandon their newly acquired freedom and return to a caregiving role. As the clinician involves these family members in the treatment process, attention to their resources as well as the stressors that are impacting each family member is essential to the effective application of the Family Based Treatment model. Families that had a workable problem-solving style premorbidly will access these intact resources and, in spite of their pain, begin to accommodate to their changed family member. Families that were conflicted and chaotic premorbidly will continue to show those same behaviors and will surely tax the clinician's creative strategizing abilities.

Developmental Disability

Families that have been raising their child with a disability since childhood will be experienced differently by the clinician. One cannot help empathizing with the pain and grief of the family with a newly injured family member. On the other hand, families that have been dealing with disability for years are often expected to have adjusted to the problem even though this may be unrealistic and may not elicit the same natural concern from the professional community. Nevertheless, it is critical for the clinician to remember that developmental transitions usually remind the family, once again, that their loved one is not "normal" and that they now have another set of issues to deal with. What kind of job, if any, will the emerging adult be able to secure? How will he/she deal with relationships and sexuality? Is independent living possible, and, if so, how much involvement should parents have? What will happen when the support systems that are readily available until age twenty-one are no longer accessible? What will happen when parents, if they are the caregivers, become ill and/or too old to care for their adult family member? And, even though the young adult and his/her parents may be well aware that handicaps are made, not born, what will happen when parents are no longer available to smooth over the anguish created by a society that has not yet learned this important fact? These and other questions may disrupt the family of the young adult as the launching years begin.

The clinician must deal with yet another factor that compounds the treatment problems associated with launching. Many families have spent twenty years or more struggling to maintain their appropriate role as parents of their child. A major part of this struggle has taken place in the offices and classrooms of the specialists that have served their child. They have heard the message from some of these professionals: "You are a problem and are not welcome. Your child would be doing well if it weren't for you." Professionals don't actually say this, of course, but parents may hear this unfortunate message. Each professional encounter has added another layer of protection to the parent-child dyad unless the family was fortunate early on to have encountered a professional who helped empower the parents in their appropriate role. The clinician that wants to involve the family in treatment during the launching phase may experience this parental protection as hostility and will need to employ reflective listening and an extra measure of respect before family members can begin to trust that their participation is really desired. Family members that appear to be "overprotective" must be enlisted on the team so that their love for their young adults is accessed and their consultative expertise is effectively utilized for change. The young adult who is moving toward independence will do so more successfully if family support and assistance is an integral part of the process. An understanding of the launching stage of family development as it occurs for all families and as it impacts families experiencing disability will help the clinician involve the family in the assessment and treatment of speech language change.

Aging Parent-Adult Interaction

During the later years stage, family interaction changes as the aging process begins to affect marital relationships, physical abilities, and the financial stability of the aging family member. The later years are a time of continuing growth and change for many individuals while steady decline and physical difficulties characterize the lives of others. Death marks the final exit of family members from the intergenerational spiral just as birth marked the individual's entrance into the family. Death, however, does not necessarily eliminate the influence of the individual who has had a unique impact on the family as it has evolved over time.

Changing marital relationships impact older adults in a number of ways. Retirement creates shifts in relationships that are easily accommodated by couples who enjoy role flexibility. These couples look forward to their retirement years and anticipate increased freedom to enjoy one another and leisure activities. Couples who are not accustomed to role flexibility will experience a period of adjustment when retirement occurs if the retired person feels bereft of responsibility while the homemaker feels that her territory has been invaded by her ever-present spouse. When retirement plans are destroyed by a debilitating stroke, heart attack, or other disease a severe developmental disruption occurs. When a spouse dies, the associated stress experienced by his life long partner is the most serious of any stressor of the later years (McCubbin & Dahl, 1985).

Physical changes that are a natural part of aging vary in impact for older adults, but each person becomes aware of a gradual decline in physical abilities. Most adjust quite easily to these normal body changes while others require frequent medical intervention.

Financial stability is critical to successful aging, but the widening gap between those who are financially stable and those whose means are sparse reflects the economic disparity evident in the wider culture. When finances are inadequate and family financial support is not available, the older adult is unable to age gracefully. Poverty and isolation are serious extenuating circumstances for many elderly persons, particularly females who outlive their male peers, and the influence of family may be felt by its absence. The clinician is likely to encounter people from a variety of life circumstances, all of whom are dealing with the disabling effects of a communicative disorder.

Any or all of the changes during the later years activate the younger generations who must now join in the decision-making process relative to their older family members. Spouses, adult children and their spouses, grandchildren, brothers, and sisters are essential members of the habilitative team as plans are made to maximize communicative competence. In the unfortunate event that the older adult has no family members available to participate in treatment, friends, acquaintances, and professional staff in long-term care facilities can be enlisted to help develop an understanding of functional language needs and to participate in the development of appropriate interventions.

When it is clear that speech-language treatment will not enhance the well-being of the aging adult and that change is not realistically possible, the ethical clinician will inform the family and/or caregiving institution of this fact and offer suggestions for alternative activities that may make the loved ones last months as comfortable as possible.

The later years stage of the family life cycle continue to be filled with complex changes that interface with the ever-evolving changes experienced by other family members. The interactive behaviors of family members as this stage evolves can be accessed, supported, and altered to assist in the enhancement of communicative strategies as speech-language treatment proceeds.

LAUNCHING AND LATER YEARS CASE STUDIES

Speech-Language Problems Associated with Mental Retardation

The launching transition can be very stressful for the individual and family of the person who is mentally retarded. The grieving process is reawakened as the family is confronted with a new set of issues. All families are faced with new tasks during the launching stage but usually with the knowledge that the child's full independence is possible and with the expectation that it will be achieved. However, the parents of a young adult who is mentally retarded, are likely to experience stress and isolation during the launching transition that is second only to that experienced at the time of the original diagnosis (Wikler, et al., 1983; Suelzle & Keenan, 1981).

Until now, school placement and support had been a major focus of the family and the loss of this management assistance can be a difficult and seemingly insurmountable challenge for many parents (Long, in press). In addition, the adult social service system presents a confusing array of possibilities that the family may not understand or know how to access. The family is often forced to become the case manager for their adult child. If they have been encouraged in this role since their child's early years, they will be accustomed to problem solving and will have the confidence and ability to meet the task at hand. If their parental role has been gradually usurped by well-meaning professionals, they are likely to flounder precariously as this management task is handed over to them. The family's search for services or a rehabilitation counselor's referral may bring the launching individual and family to the speech-language pathologist's door.

Mrs. Stevens, Bob's mother, called the speech-language clinician soon after her son's twenty-third birthday. Bob had just been accepted by a sheltered workshop following a vocational rehabilitation assessment and was having difficulty following directions and communicating with supervisors and co-workers. The workshop supervisor suggested that speech-language treatment might facilitate Bob's communicative competence as he was integrated into the work situation.

Mrs. Stevens said that she didn't know exactly why the referral had been made because she understood Bob perfectly and wondered aloud if the people at the workshop were treating her son fairly. The clinician suggested that since the mother was able to communicate successfully with her son it would be very helpful if she could accompany him to the first session. Mother readily agreed.

During the telephone convening conversation, the clinician learned that Bob was a mentally retarded adult living at home with his mother and father and that his two older sisters were launched and lived some distance from the parental home. The clinician asked Mrs. Stevens to invite her husband to accompany her and Bob to the session. She replied that he would probably come but would not say much because he usually left these things up to her. Appreciation was expressed to Mrs. Stevens for inviting her husband and she was assured that it was fine if he did not want to talk much. The clinician added that he probably would not speak much unless he had something important to share. It was hoped that this statement would relieve Mrs. Stevens of the worry that her "quiet" husband would be pressured into contributing when he was unwilling to do so. Since Mr. Stevens was recently retired and Mrs. Stevens was a homemaker, a daytime appointment was arranged immediately following the end of Bob's work day.

Application to Adults and Their Families 185

The family arrived at the appointed time. Bob, a large gregarious man, greeted the clinician with an affable smile and immediately reached out to shake the clinician's hand. The clinician introduced herself, chatted a bit, and asked Bob to introduce her to his parents. This act immediately underscored Bob's status as an emerging adult who would be the primary focus of the clinician's work while simultaneously indicating the importance of his parents as consultants to the treatment process. Mom smiled pleasantly and following her introduction to the clinician instructed Bob to remove his jacket because "It's hot in here." Bob readily complied and the clinician led the family to the treatment room where the introductions were completed. Mr. Stevens, a quiet person possessing the same size and apparent physical strength of his son, looked glum and decidedly unhappy as he seated himself in the room. His quiet demeanor was a powerful contrast to the animated discussion taking place between Mrs. Stevens and Bob as they discussed the temperature of the room and the advisability of wearing jackets and coats.

The clinician noted to herself that Bob was wearing a hearing aid, a fact that she had failed to learn during the initial telephone conversation. She also noted that Bob's speech was characterized by difficulty with sibilant sounds and that his rapid rate of speech added to his unintelligibility.

The family interview and the accompanying spontaneous enactments clearly underscored Mrs. Stevens' belief that she understood Bob perfectly. The clinician was able to understand most of Bob's utterances and whenever she appeared to be somewhat quizzical, Mrs. Stevens willingly and readily interpreted. Each time this happened, Bob was asked if his mother's interpretation was correct and only once did he have to alter what she had said. No overt communication was observed between Mr. Stevens and his son.

Bob was asked to read words and sentences to assess his articulation further. As Mr. Stevens observed this process, his unhappy facial expression was replaced by a look of curiosity and amusement. The clinician hypothesized that this may have been one of the few times that he had participated in a visit to a professional's office relative to his son's habilitative program.

The clinician explained her findings as she learned the characteristics of Bob's speech. She discussed the fact that he had a mild, inconsistent hypernasality; a number of inconsistent errors on consonants; and a consistent oral distortion of sibilant sounds, most notably /s/. Mrs. Stevens reiterated that she understood Bob perfectly and the clinician responded that this was absolutely true, but apparently people who did not know Bob as well as she did had some difficulty communicating with him. Mr. Stevens then spoke for the first time saying that, "Even people who know him well have trouble." The clinician asked if that was sometimes the case for him and he replied, "Yes." Mrs. Stevens offered the suggestion that treatment might be good so that other people could understand him, but that they would also have to try a little harder and learn to be more patient with Bob. The clinician responded by asserting that this was a good point and that a meeting with the people at the workshop might facilitate a better understanding of the difficulties experienced in that setting. Mrs. Stevens was assured that she would also be part of the meeting, as would Bob, and she offered to try to set something up.

Data gathering continued as the clinician questioned Bob about his hearing loss and the effects of this on his communication with other people. He said that he often had difficulty understanding other people, particularly when the TV was on. In a quiet room during face to face contact, he "can understand everything." The clinician asked Bob to get an audiological evaluation and gave him instructions for making the appointment. Mr. Stevens said that he would see that Bob had transportation to the appointment.

Tentative times for a workshop meeting were discussed, exchange of information forms signed, and the first session ended. The clinician noted that Mr. Stevens seemed relaxed and less glum than at the start of the session and asked him if he too would be interested in attending a meeting at the sheltered workshop. His reply, "I suppose so," was viewed as positive and the family departed the first session.

The results of the audiological examination revealed a moderate-to-severe sensorineural loss for the right ear and a profound hearing loss in the left ear. The hearing aid worn in the right ear produced a speech reception threshold at 20 dB HL and a speech discrimination score of 76 percent.

At the beginning of the second session, the clinician reaffirmed Mrs. Stevens' ability to communicate effectively with her son and asked the parents if they were willing to go along with Bob's desire for improvement since this might help him communicate with his peers in his new job situation. Mr. and Mrs. Stevens agreed and said that a meeting had been arranged at the sheltered workshop to further assess Bob's communicative difficulties.

Speech-language treatment included the development of communication strategies such as slower speech, exaggerated articulation, increased effort, and increased pitch as well as attempts to improve his production of specific consonants. Bob explained to his father that he could understand him better if they faced each other when they talked and if Dad would "SPEAK UP." The clinician conducted the sessions as she would have conducted individual sessions but with the parents present and participating as they wished. Both Mr. and Mrs. Stevens became increasingly comfortable asking questions and making suggestions. A turning point seemed to occur when Mr.

Stevens suggested that he and Bob could probably talk better if the TV were turned off.

The network meeting at the sheltered workshop identified the problems Bob had communicating with peers when the environment was noisy, and the decision was made to move him to a job in a quieter environment. There he would associate with only two other people and would be less overwhelmed as he attempted to slow his rate of speech and implement his newly acquired articulation strategies. Everyone present was asked to pay attention to Bob's communication and to encourage Bob as he made an effort to communicate more effectively. The friendly, cooperative style shown by everyone at the meeting pleased Bob and his parents.

Treatment continued for six months. At the end of the second month, Mr. and Mrs. Stevens felt that they understood what was going on and decided to go out for coffee while Bob was in his session. This appropriate differentiation underscored Bob's independence from his parents. The parents felt that they didn't need to be "watching over him every minute" since he was already twenty-three years old.

Maximum change occurred as a result of Bob's efforts, the cooperation of his parents, and the reinforcement received from the staff of the sheltered workshop. Mrs. Stevens remarked that even she found it easier to talk to her son. Treatment terminated with the understanding that Bob would call the clinician if he decided he needed further help. His speech was not perfect, but significant changes had occurred. He was interacting more effectively with his father and had received the "Worker of the Month" award at the sheltered workshop.

Consultation Related To Aphasia

In other cases, clinicians who work systemically are

Application to Adults and Their Families 189

likely to be called upon by families for one or two-session consultations. Families who request this are not seeking assessment and treatment in the usual sense but want the speech-language pathologist's opinion about a communicative problem and/or suggestions for ways to improve interaction with a family member having a communicative disorder. Termination of services is expected after the number of agreed-upon sessions has been completed.

A consultation session was requested by the family of Mrs. Alban, an 85 year old woman who lived in a nursing home. Her family included three adult children and their spouses. All lived within fifty miles of the nursing home and visited her on a regular basis. The clinician was contacted by one of the adult children and asked to meet with Mrs. Alban and her family in the nursing home to discuss how communication with her could be enhanced. Mrs. Alban's family believed that she wanted to interact with them but could not "move her mouth correctly" to do so.

We met with Mrs. Alban and her family in the sunroom of the nursing home. Family members present included her two daughters and her son and his wife. Mrs. Alban was in a wheel chair repeating, "wishy- wishy" in a quiet voice looking at nothing or no one in particular. We watched as family members spoke with her and observed that nearly every interaction was a question (eg., Do you know who's here? Who am I, mom? Did you remember to take your pill? What day is it? Did you have breakfast? What did you eat? Did you eat it all? Were you able to eat today? Did the nurses help you? Do you know where we are?) or commands (eg., C'mon mom, you've got to try. Try my name; say Mike. Today is Monday; you say it. Say Monday, mom. Look at me; watch my mouth. Watch!).

After observing the attempts of family members to interact with Mrs. Alban, we made a special point of neither asking questions nor giving commands as we initially spoke with her. Rather, we attempted to make only statements. Mrs. Alban did not actually respond to these any differently than she did to the questions and commands of her children. In fact, if anything, she seemed more pleased to hear her children's voices than ours.

We listened as family members gave their perspective of the problem. They sensed the gravity of the problem even though they continued to use terms implying that their mother's communicative ability would improve. As we talked more and observed one another interact with Mrs. Alban, it became clear that change in her expressive communicative behavior was not a realistic goal. We began asking for information about the adult children's common family as they were growing up, their mother's interests, their father's characteristics, and their mother's role in the family. What evolved was a mini-history of the family with each adult child being eager to relay interactions that he or she had had with mother. They described their mother as a key person in the home as they were growing up and one who had made most of the decisions, done most of the disciplining, and who was primarily responsible for the care of the children. At this point we returned to our discussion of the severity of Mrs. Alban's communication problem. We suggested that they talk about childhood and family experiences as they interact with their mother in order to remind her, to the extent possible, of past events and to provide communicative input that she might enjoy. We framed the latter suggestion in terms of the life review (Lewis & Butler, 1974) that is very meaningful when done by and with older persons as they near the end of life. We pointed out that their mother responded more positively to their voices than she did to ours and that if they were to speak slowly while touching her hand or arm (which they had already been doing) she might appreciate these memories more than attempts to orient her and "demonstrate" her understanding.

The consultation session lasted one and one-half hours. The family members expressed appreciation for our help and seemed satisfied that they were doing all that they could for their mother. A follow-up session was scheduled to be held in two months. When working with aging persons whose communication is severely disordered, a family consultation session is likely to help families establish communication strategies that assist them as they anticipate the impending death of their family member. The aging person will also benefit from the loving concern offered by the people who mean the most to him or her.

SUMMARY

Significant developmental changes occur during the adult years. The launching family must adjust to their emerging young-adult member who is establishing independence. When injury or illness disrupts this process, the impact on the family is often severe. Families must also accommodate to their young-adult member who has been developmentally disabled since childhood as his/her role in the larger society is defined.

Older family members often enjoy active and productive lives and are supportive members of their children and grandchildren's treatment teams. Other aging persons may be forced to deal with illness and disability. Family support is critical to the well-being of these individuals and the speech-language pathologist should enlist the family's help as treatment is planned and implemented. When family members are unavailable, friends and professional staff may be recruited to provide communication reinforcement in the older person's natural context.

BIBLIOGRAPHY

Anderson S., Russell, C. & Schumm, W. (1983). Perceived marital quality and family life cycle categories: A further analysis. *Journal of Marriage and the Family, 45,* 127-139.

Andrews, J. & Andrews, M. (1986a). A short-term family systems approach to speech-language treatment as a supplement to school-based services. *Seminars in Speech and Language, 7,* 407-414.

Andrews, J. & Andrews, M. (1986b). A family-based systemic model for speech-language services. *Seminars in Speech and Language, 7,* 359-365.

Andrews, M. (1986). Application of family therapy techniques to the treatment of language disorders. *Seminars In Speech and Language, 7,* 347-358.

Bateson, G. (1979). *Mind and nature.* New York: Dutton.

Benjamin, A. (1981). *The helping interview.* Boston: Houghton Mifflin.

Burr, W. (1972). Role transitions: A reformulation of theory. *Journal of Marriage and the Family, 34,* 407-416.

Carrow-Woolfolk, E. & Lynch, J. (1982). *An integrative approach to language disorders in children.* New York: Grune & Stratton.

Carter, E.A. & McGoldrick, M. (1980). The family life cycle and family therapy: An overview. In E.A. Carter and M. McGoldrick (Eds.), *The family life cycle: A framework for family therapy* (pp. 3-20). New York: Gardner Press, Inc.

Dell, P. F. (1982). Beyond homeostasis: Toward a concept of coherence. *Family Process, 21,* 21-41.

DePompei, R. (1987). A systems approach to understanding CHI family functioning. *Cognitive Rehabilitation,* March/April,1987, 6-10.

deShazer, S. (1985). *Keys to solution in brief therapy.* New York: W.W. Norton.

deShazer, S. (1982). Some conceptual distinctions are more useful than others. *Family Process, 21,* 71-84.

Duvall, E. M. (1977). *Family development.* (5th Ed.). Philadelphia: Lippincott.

Dyer, E. (1963). Parenthood as crisis: A restudy. *Marriage and Family Living, 25,* 196-201.

Epstein, N. & Bishop, D. (1981). Problem centered systems therapy of the family. In A. S. Gurman & D. P. Kniskern (Eds.), *Handbook of family therapy* (pp. 444-482). New York: Brunner/Mazel.

Fisch, R., Weakland, J. H. & Segal, L. (1982). *The tactics of change.* San Francisco: Jossey Bass.

Fleuridas, C., Nelson, T. and Rosenthal, D. (1986). The evolution of circular questions: Training family therapists. *Journal of Marital and Family Therapy, 12,* 113-127.

Fortier, L. & Wanlass, R. L. (1984). Family crisis following the diagnosis of a handicapped child. *Family Relations, 33,* 3-24.

Frassinelli, L., Superior, K. & Meyers, J. (1983). A consultation model for speech and language services. *ASHA, 25,* 25-30.

Bibliography

Garbee, F. (1982). The speech-language pathologist as a member of the educational team. In R.J. Van Hattum (Ed.) *Speech-Language Programming in the Schools* (pp.72-115). Springfield, IL: Charles C. Thomas Publisher.

Glenn, N. (1975). Psychological well-being in the post-parental stage: Some evidence from national surveys. *Journal of Marriage and the Family, 37*, 105-110.

Goetz, N. (1982). Parental perspectives and concerns. *Seminars in Speech, Language and Hearing, 3*, 274-279.

Hahn, E. (1979). Directed home training program for infants with cleft lip and palate. In K.R. Bzoch (Ed.), *Communicative disorders related to cleft lip and palate* (pp. 311-317). Boston: Little, Brown and Company.

Haley, J. (1987). *Problem solving therapy.* San Francisco: Jossey-Bass.

Haley, J. (1973). *Uncommon therapy: The psychiatric techniques of Milton H. Erickson, M.D.* New York: Norton.

Hofstadter, D. (1979). *Godel, Escher, Bach: An eternal golden braid.* New York: Basic Books.

Johnson, B., McGonigel, M. & Kaufmann, R. (Eds.) (1989). *Guidelines and recommended practices for the individualized family service plan.* Chapel Hill, N.C.: NEC*TAS.

Keeney, B. P. (1983). *The aesthetics of change.* New York: The Guilford Press.

LeMasters, E. (1957). Parenthood as crisis. *Marriage and Family Living, 19*, 352-355.

Lewis. M. & Butler, R. (1974). Life review therapy. *Geriatrics, 29*, 165-173.

Long, G. (in press). Introduction. In Long, G. & Harvey, M. (Eds.), *Facilitating the transition of deaf adolescents: Focus on families.* (pp. 1-9). Manuscript submitted for publication.

Luterman, D. (1984). *Counseling the communicatively disordered and their families.* Boston: Little, Brown & Co.

Manolson, A., (1985). *It takes two to talk: A Hanen early language parent guide book.* Toronto: Hanen Early Language Resource Centre.

Madanes, C. (1981). *Strategic family therapy.* San Francisco: Jossey Bass.

McCubbin, H. & Dahl. B. (1985). *Family and marriage: Individuals and lifecycles.* New York: John Wiley & Sons.

Minuchin, S. (1974). *Families and family therapy.* Cambridge: Harvard University Press.

Moores, D. F. (1985). Educational programs and services for hearing impaired children: Issues and options. In Powell, F., Finitzo-Hieber, T., Friel-Patti, S. & Henderson, D. (Eds.) *Education of the hearing impaired child.* (pp. 3-20). San Diego: College Hill Press.

Moses, K. (1985). Dynamic intervention with families. In: *Hearing-impaired children and youth with developmental disabilities: An interdisciplinary foundation for service.* (pp. 82-98) Washington, DC: Gallaudet College Press.

Neidecker, E. (1987). *School programs in speech-language: Organization and management.* Englewood Cliffs: Prentice Hall.

Northern, J. L. & Downs, M. P. (1974). *Hearing in children.* Baltimore: Williams and Wilkins.

O'Hanlon, W. H. & Weiner-Davis, M. (1989). *In search of solutions.* New York: W. W. Norton, & Co.

Rogers, C. (1965). *Client centered therapy.* Boston: Houghton Mifflin.

Rollin, W. J. (1987). *The psychology of communication disorders in individuals and their families.* Englewood Cliffs, New Jersey: Prentice-Hall, Inc.

Rollins, B. & Feldman, H. (1970). Marital satisfaction over the family life cycle. *Journal of Marriage and the Family, 32,* 20-28.

Schlesinger, H.S. (1985). Deafness, mental health, and language. In F. Powell, T. Finitzo-Hieber, S. Friel-Patti, and D. Henderson (Eds.), *Education of the hearing impaired child* (pp. 103-116). San Diego: College-Hill Press.

Schwartz, L. (1982). Social services for the family with a cleft palate child. *Seminars in Speech, Language and Hearing, 3,* 268-273.

Scott, S. (1984). Mobilization: A natural resource of the family. In J. C. Hansen & E. I. Coppersmith (Eds.), *Families with handicapped members* (pp. 98-110). Rockville, MD: Aspen Systems Corporation.

Seibel, N. (1987a). A parent's perspective. *The ACPA/CPF Newsletter* (pp. 1-2). American Cleft Palate Association: Pittsburgh, PA.

Seibel, N. (1987b). Untitled. Unpublished manuscript.

Simon, F., Stierlin, H. & Wynne, L. (1985). *The language of family therapy: A systemic vocabulary and sourcebook.* New York: Family Process Press.

Snow, C. (1984). Foreword. *Topics in Language Disorders, 4*, pp.v.

Solomon, M. A. (1973). A developmental conceptual premise for family therapy. *Family Process, 12*, 179-188.

Spanbock, P. (1987). Understanding head injury from the families' perspective. *Cognitive Rehabilitation*. March/April, 12-14.

Suelzle, M., & Keenan, V. (1981). Changes in family support networks over the life cycle of mentally retarded persons. *American Journal of Mental Deficiency, 86*, 267-274.

Superior, K. & Lelchook, A. (1986). Family participation in school-based programs. *Seminars in Speech and Language, 7*, 395-404.

Tomm, K. (1984). One perspective on the Milan systemic approach: Part I. Overview of development, theory and practice. *Journal of Marital and Family Therapy, 10*, 113-125.

Tomm, K. (1988). Interventive interviewing: Part III. Intending to ask circular, strategic, or reflexive questions. *Family Process, 27*, 1-15.

Vander Zanden, J. W. (1989). *Human development*. New York: Alfred A. Knopf.

Van Riper, C. (1954). *Speech correction: Principles and Methods*. Englewood Cliffs, NJ: Prentice-Hall.

Watzlawick, P., Weakland, J., & Fisch, R. (1974). *Change: Principles of problem formation and problem resolution*. New York: W. W. Norton & Co.

Wilcox, M. J. (1989). Delivering communication-based services to infants, toddlers, and their families: Approaches and models. *Topics in Language Disorders, 10,* 68-79.

Wikler, L., Wasow, M., & Hatfield, E. (1983). Looking for strengths in families of developmentally disabled children. *Social Work,* July/August, 313-315.

Williams, S. C. (1986). Family-focused treatment: A speech-language pathologists role in a home-based parent training program. *Seminars in Speech and Language, 7,* 383-393.

INDEX

Accommodation, 42-43, 124, 125-126
Adolescence
    case involving, 54-56, 75-77, 162-167
    issues of, 155-160
Adulthood
    case involving, 184-188, 189-191
    issues of, 175-183
Anderson, S., 175
Andrews, J., 12, 13, 18
Andrews, M., 12, 13, 18, 89
Aphasia, case involving, 189-191
Articulation, case involving, 51-54, 160-167, 167-169
Assessing effectiveness
    assignments, 65-66
Assessment
    of treatment effectiveness, 65-66, 78-82
    results of, 108-109
Assignments, 47, 61-69
    assessing effectiveness type, 65-66
    clinician intent, 63, 66
    creation of, 52, 55, 58, 61
    delivering to family, 66, 104-106
    enactment of, 81-82
    idiosyncratic nature of, 27-28, 150-151
    intervention type, 64-65
    noticing type, 62-64
    review of, 79-81
Attending, in counseling, 91

Bateson, G., 1
Benjamin, A., 92
Bishop, D., 16, 17, 19, 20
Both/and perspective, 8-9
Burns, M., v.
Burr, W., 119
Butler, R., 190

Carrow-Woolfolk, E., 132
Carter, E., 117, 118, 155, 175
Cause-effect change, 7, 12

Child-rearing, 156-157
Clarification, 92-94
    example of, 92-94
Cleft palate, case involving, 134-141
Closure, during grief process, 114
Compliance, 5, 15
Compliment, use of, 67, 104-105
Consultation
    case involving, 188-191
    with family, 87, 188-189
    with grandparents, 122-123
    with professionals, 88, 110
Convening, 29-35
    sample conversation, 31-33
    use of language, 33-34
Cooperation, 5, 25-28, 107-108, 126-127
Counseling
    integrating into treatment, 89, 106-110
    techniques, 89-106
    use of in communicative disorders, 15-16
Creative strategizing, 51, 61, 103, 104, 105

Dahl, B., 181
Defining the system, 30-31, 162-163
Dell, P., 13
Denial, 109-110, 113-114
DePompei, R., 179
deShazer, S., 2, 7, 38, 104, 107
Developmental
    disability, 119, 179-181
    case involving, 184-188
    disruptions, 119-120
    factors of adulthood, 175-177
    factors of early childhood, 118-123
    factors of middle childhood and adolescence, 153-154
    stages, 117
Downs, M. P., 147
Duvall, E., 117
Dyer, E., 119
Dysarthria, case involving, 75-77

Early childhood, 119
　case involving, 51-54, 56-58, 72-75, 124-134, 134-141, 143-147, 148-153
　issues of, 118-123
Either/or perspective, 8-9
Empathic listening, 109-110
Empowerment
　of families, 26-27, 44, 105, 135, 155
　of parents, 120, 147-148
Enactment, use of, 49, 81-82, 126, 127, 185
Epstein, N., 16, 17, 19, 20
Evaluation, see Testing
Extended family, 30, 122-123, 159, 172-174
　case involving, 148-153, 170-173

Family
　agreement/disagreement, 42-43, 124
　cooperation, 105
　concerns, 25-27
　developmental stages, 117-118
　expertise, 24
　expression of emotion, 24-25, 107
　interactive patterns, 17, 51, 54, 56
　participation, 44-47
　perspective, 37, 38-40
　resources, 8, 15, 50-51, 63, 105-106, 127, 144, 171-172
First order change, 77
Fisch, R., 2, 77
Feldman, H., 119, 175
Fleuridas, C., 99
Frassinelli, L., 6
Focusing outward, 113-114
Fortier, L., 112, 114

Garbee, F., 6
Glenn, N., 175
Goals
　setting, 49-59
　review of, 78-79
Goetz, N., 135
Grandparents, as consultants, 122

Grieving
　as a stage, 113
　example of, 134-135
　process, 111-116
　stages, 112-114
　variations in, 114-116

Hahn, E., 135
Haley, J., 2, 103, 104, 117
Hatfield, E., 183
Hearing-impairment, case involving, 148-153, 184-188
Hierarchical structure, 20, 40, 50
Hofstadter, D., 38

Impact, during grief process, 112
Individual family service plans, 124
Intent, of clinician, 63
Interaction
　aging parent-adult, 181-183
　attending to, 72-78
　extended family, 159-160
　parent-child, 156-157
　parent-young adult, 177-178
　peer, 158-159
　sibling, 157-158
Interactive
　behaviors, 19-21
　patterns, 9-10, 40-41, 102-103
　sequences, 51, 54, 56
　style, 41
　uniqueness, 27
Intergenerational
　conflict, 160
　differences, 123
　issues, 176-177
Intervention assignment, 64-65
Interviewing techniques, application of, 108
Isomorphism, 37-38, 67, 127

Johnson, B., 124
Joining
　use of, 31, 38-39, 50
　process of, 90-91

Index

Kaufmann, R., 124
Keenan, V., 183
Keeney, B. P., 2, 71

Labeling behaviors, 9-10
Language,
    case involving, 56-58, 72-75, 124-134, 169-170, 170-173
    use of, 33-34
Launching, developmental stage of, 155, 177-178, 180, 183
Lelchook, A., 6
LeMasters, E., 119
Lewis, M., 190
Linear
    model, 5-6
    paradigm, 7
Linking, to other professionals, 87-88
Long, G., 183
Luterman, D., 113
Lynch, J., 132

Madanes, C., 103
Manolson, A., 6
McCubbin H., 181
McGoldrick, M., 117, 118, 155, 175
McGonigel, M., 124
Meyers, J., 6
Minuchin, S., 2, 90, 98
Mobilization points, 41-42, 46, 50, 52, 54, 57, 126
Moores, D. F., 147
Moses, K., 111-113, 119

Negotiating boundaries, 156-157
Neidecker, E., 6
Nelson, T., 99
Neutral questioning, 99-101
Northern, J., 147
Noticing assignments, 62-64

O'Hanlon, W. H., 2, 12
One truth to many truths, 7-8

Paradigm
    linear, 7
    shift, 6-14
    systemic, 7
Phonological disorder, case involving, 79-82, 160-169
Polyocular view, 7-8
Problem focus, 10-12

Reflective listening, 94-97
    example of, 96-97
Reinforcement, 45
Resources of the family, see Family
Restatement, use of, 94
Roles
    of parents, 120-122
    of professionals, 15
Rogers, C., 91, 94
Rollin, W. J., 178
Rollins, B., 119, 175
Rosenthal, D., 99
Russell, C., 175

Scheduling, of families, 34-35
Schlesinger, H., 147
Schumm, W., 175
Schwartz, L., 135
Scott, S., 42
Second order change, 77
Segal, L., 2
Seibel, N., 136, 141
Sibling relationships, 157-158
Simon, F., 90
Simple actions, 71-78
Snow, C., 123
Solo-parent family, 121
Solomon, M., 117
Solution focus, 10-12
Spanbock, P., 112
Stages of crisis and loss, 112-114
Standardized tests, 47-48
Stierlin, H., 90
Stop and say, 82
Strategic family therapists, 2
Stuttering, case involving, 143-149
Suezle, M., 183

Summarizing, 98, 125
   statements, 98
Superior, K., 6
System transformation, 12-14
Systemic
   clinician, 6-7
   perspectives, 10, 99
   principles, 16-21

Task assignments, 104-106
Termination of treatment, 85-87
Testing, 44-45, 47-48
   with family participation, 44-47, 127-128, 164
Tomm, K., 2, 12, 99
Tracking
   example of, 99-101
   interactive patterns, 98-103, 126
   spontaneous enactments of, 102
Transactional patterns, 19
Traumatic brain injury, case
   involving, 54-56
Treatment model
   traditional-individual, 5-6, 37-38, 61, 71
   systemic, 14-16, 37-38, 61, 71

Unit of treatment, 14-15

Vacation, from treatment, 86
   example of, 138
Vander Zanden, J. W., 176
Van Riper, C., 141

Wanlass, R., 112, 114
Wasow, M., 183
Watzlawick, P., 77
Weakland, J. H., 2, 77
Weiner-Davis, M., 2, 12
Wikler, L., 183
Wilcox, M. J., 165
Williams, S. C., 6
Wynne, L., 90